Cancer Precursor Conditions and their Detection

Editor

ELIZABETH K. O'DONNELL

HEMATOLOGY/ONCOLOGY CLINICS OF NORTH AMERICA

www.hemonc.theclinics.com

Consulting Editors
GEORGE P. CANELLOS
EDWARD J. BENZ JR

August 2024 • Volume 38 • Number 4

ELSEVIER

1600 John F. Kennedy Boulevard • Suite 1800 • Philadelphia, Pennsylvania, 19103-2899

http://www.theclinics.com

HEMATOLOGY/ONCOLOGY CLINICS OF NORTH AMERICA Volume 38, Number 4
August 2024 ISSN 0889-8588, ISBN 13: 978-0-443-29350-4

Editor: Stacy Eastman
Developmental Editor: Malvika Shah

Hematology/Oncology Clinics (ISSN 0889-8588) is published bimonthly by Elsevier Inc., 360 Park Avenue South, New York, NY 10010-1710. Months of issue are February, April, June, August, October, and December. Business and Editorial Offices: 1600 John F. Kennedy Blvd., Ste. 1800, Philadelphia, PA 19103–2899. Customer Service Office: 3251 Riverport Lane, Maryland Heights, MO 63043. Periodicals postage paid at New York, NY and at additional mailing offices. Subscription prices are $498.00 per year (domestic individuals), $100.00 per year (domestic students/residents), $525.00 per year (Canadian individuals), $100.00 per year (Canadian students/residents), $597.00 per year (international individuals), and $255.00 per year (international students/residents). For institutional access pricing please contact Customer Service via the contact information below. International air speed delivery is included in all *Clinics* subscription prices. All prices are subject to change without notice. **POSTMASTER:** Send address changes to *Hematology/Oncology Clinics of North America*, Elsevier Health Sciences Division, Subscription Customer Service, 3251 Riverport Lane, Maryland Heights, MO 63043. Customer Service (orders, claims, online, change of address): Elsevier Health Sciences Division, Subscription **Customer Service, 3251 Riverport Lane, Maryland Heights, MO 63043. Tel: 1-800-654-2452 (U.S. and Canada); 314-447-8871 (outside U.S. and Canada). Fax: 314-447-8029. E-mail: journalscustomerservice-usa@elsevier.com (for print support); journalsonlinesupport-usa@elsevier.com (for online support).**

Reprints. For copies of 100 or more, of articles in this publication, please contact the Commercial Reprints Department, Elsevier Inc., 360 Park Avenue South, New York, New York 10010-1710; Tel.: 212-633-3874, Fax: 212-633-3820, E-mail: reprints@elsevier.com.

Hematology/Oncology Clinics of North America is covered in *MEDLINE/PubMed (Index Medicus), EMBASE/ Excerpta Medica, and BIOSIS.*

Contributors

CONSULTING EDITORS

GEORGE P. CANELLOS, MD
William Rosenberg Professor of Medicine, Department of Medical Oncology, Dana-Farber Cancer Institute, Boston, Massachusetts, USA

EDWARD J. BENZ Jr, MD
Professor, Pediatrics, Richard and Susan Smith Professor, Medicine, Professor, Genetics, Harvard Medical School, President and CEO Emeritus, Office of the President, Dana-Farber Cancer Institute, Boston, Massachusetts, USA

EDITOR

ELIZABETH K. O'DONNELL, MD
Physician, Department of Medical Oncology, Director of Early Detection and Prevention, Dana-Farber Cancer Institute, Assistant Professor of Medicine, Harvard Medical School, Boston, Massachusetts, USA

AUTHORS

BRITTANY A. BORDEN, MD
Resident Physician, Department of Medicine, Brigham and Women's Hospital, Boston, Massachusetts, USA

BRITTANY L. BYCHKOVSKY, MD, MSc
Assistant Professor of Medicine, Division of Cancer Genetics and Prevention, Department of Medical Oncology, Dana-Farber Cancer Institute, Harvard Medical School, Boston, Massachusetts, USA

ALLISON E.B. CHANG, MD, PhD
Fellow, Department of Medicine, Division of Hematology/Oncology, Massachusetts General Hospital, Department of Hematology/Oncology, Dana Farber Cancer Institute, Harvard Medical School, Boston, Massachusetts, USA

PIETRO DE PLACIDO, MD
Research Fellow, Department of Medical Oncology, Dana-Farber Cancer Institute, Boston, Massachusetts, USA

FLORENTIA DIMITRIOU, MD, PhD
Fellow, Department of Surgical Oncology, The University of Texas MD Anderson Cancer Center, Houston, Texas, USA; Dermatologist, Department of Dermatology, University Hospital of Zurich, University of Zurich, Zurich, Switzerland

IRENE M. GHOBRIAL, MD
Lavine Family Chair for Preventative Cancer Therapies, Dana-Farber Cancer Institute, Harvard Medical School, Boston, Massachusetts, USA

GLENN J. HANNA, MD
Department of Medical Oncology, Center for Head and Neck Oncology, Dana-Farber Cancer Institute, Assistant Professor of Medicine, Harvard Medical School, Boston, Massachusetts, USA

NICHOLAS A. HODGES, PhD
Program Director, Cancer Biomarkers Research Group, Division of Cancer Prevention, National Cancer Institute, NIH, Rockville, Maryland, USA

INDU KOHAAR, PhD
Program Director, Cancer Biomarkers Research Group, Division of Cancer Prevention, National Cancer Institute, NIH, Rockville, Maryland, USA

ASAF MAOZ, MD
Instructor, Dana-Farber Cancer Institute, Harvard Medical School, Boston, Massachusetts, USA

SARA MYERS, MD, PhD
Harvard Medical School, Brigham and Women's Hospital, Boston, Massachusetts, USA

KELLY C. NELSON, MD
Professor, Department of Dermatology, The University of Texas MD Anderson Cancer Center, Houston, Texas, USA

ELIZABETH K. O'DONNELL, MD
Physician, Department of Medical Oncology, Director of Early Detection and Prevention, Dana-Farber Cancer Institute, Assistant Professor of Medicine, Harvard Medical School, Boston, Massachusetts, USA

GIOVANNI PARMIGIANI, PhD
Professor, Department of Data Science, Dana Farber Cancer Institute, Department of Biostatistics, Harvard T.H. Chan School of Public Health, Boston, Massachusetts, USA

HEATHER A. PARSONS, MD, MPH
Assistant Professor of Medicine, Department of Medical Oncology, Dana-Farber Cancer Institute, Harvard Medical School, Boston, Massachusetts, USA; Broad Institute of MIT and Harvard, Cambridge, Massachusetts, USA

ALEXANDRA L. POTTER, BS
Clinical Research Coordinator, Division of Thoracic Surgery, Department of Surgery, Massachusetts General Hospital, Boston, Massachusetts, USA

NICOLETTE J. RODRIGUEZ, MD, MPH
Instructor, Division of Gastroenterology, Hepatology and Endoscopy, Brigham and Women's Hospital, Harvard Medical School, Division of Cancer Genetics and Prevention, Boston, Massachusetts, USA

VIKRANT V. SAHASRABUDDHE, MBBS, MPH, DrPH
Deputy Chief and Program Director, Breast and Gynecologic Cancer Research Group, Division of Cancer Prevention, National Cancer Institute, National Institutes of Health, Rockville, Maryland, USA

LECIA V. SEQUIST, MD, MPH
Professor, Department of Medicine, Division of Hematology/Oncology, Massachusetts General Hospital, Harvard Medical School, Boston, Massachusetts, USA

SUDHIR SRIVASTAVA, PhD, MPH
Senior Scientific Officer, Chief, Cancer Biomarkers Research Group, Division of Cancer Prevention, National Cancer Institute, NIH, Rockville, Maryland, USA

SAPNA SYNGAL, MD, MPH
Director of Research, Center for Cancer Genetics and Prevention, Co-Director, Centers for Early Detection and Interception, Dana Farber Cancer Institute, Boston, Massachusetts, USA

MADISON M. TAYLOR, BSA
Medical Student, John P. and Kathrine G. McGovern Medical School, The University of Texas Health Science Center, Research Fellow, Department of Dermatology, The University of Texas MD Anderson Cancer Center, Houston, Texas, USA

ALESSANDRO VILLA, DDS, PhD, MPH
Chief, Oral Medicine, Oral Oncology and Dentistry, Miami Cancer Institute, Baptist Health South Florida, Professor, Herbert Wertheim College of Medicine, Florida International University, Miami, Florida, USA

LAURA E.G. WARREN, MD
Harvard Medical School, Assistant Professor, Department of Radiation Oncology, Dana-Farber Cancer Institute, Boston, Massachusetts, USA

WILLIAM N. WILLIAM Jr, MD
Medical Oncologist, National Leader, Thoracic Oncology Program, Grupo Oncocl'nicas Grupo Oncocl'nicas, São Paulo, São Paulo, Brazil

CHI-FU JEFFREY YANG, MD
Associate Professor, Thoracic Surgeon, Harvard Medical School, Division of Thoracic Surgery, Department of Surgery, Massachusetts General Hospital, Boston, Massachusetts, USA

MATTHEW B. YURGELUN, MD
Director, Lynch Syndrome Center, Dana-Farber Cancer Institute, Associate Professor of Medicine, Harvard Medical School, Boston, Massachusetts, USA

Contents

> Strategies for early detection and interception of cancer are based on 2 synergistic elements: proactive search for asymptomatic cancer, pre-cancer, or cancer predisposition and proactive disruption of cancer evolution. Benefits and harms of both these elements will vary widely depending on the screened populations, the types of cancers targeted, the detection modalities, and the health care delivery approaches following diagnosis. This article attempts to identify common elements that can inform the evaluation of alternative strategies across many of these scenarios.

> Precursor diseases of multiple myeloma (MM) are monoclonal gammopathy of uncertain significance and smoldering MM. While it is well known that a percentage of those affected by these conditions will progress to MM, it is difficult to predict who will progress and when, and guidelines for screening for these conditions are lacking. Moreover, there are various models for risk stratification, though there are ongoing efforts to improve these models in order to predict who may benefit from treatment. Finally, there are various clinical trials, both past and ongoing, expanding the scope of possible treatment options for precursor diseases.

> Recent advances in lung cancer treatment have led to dramatic improvements in 5-year survival rates. And yet, lung cancer remains the leading cause of cancer-related mortality, in large part, because it is often diagnosed at an advanced stage, when cure is no longer possible. Lung cancer screening (LCS) is essential for intercepting the disease at an earlier stage. Unfortunately, LCS has been poorly adopted in the United States, with less than 5% of eligible patients being screened nationally. This article will describe the data supporting LCS, the obstacles to LCS implementation, and the promising opportunities that lie ahead.

> Cervical cancer, caused due to oncogenic types of human papillomavirus (HPV), is a leading preventable cause of cancer morbidity and mortality globally. Chronic, persistent HPV infection–induced cervical precursor

lesions, if left undetected and untreated, can progress to invasive cancer. Cervical cancer screening approaches have evolved from cytology (Papanicolaou test) to highly sensitive HPV-based molecular methods and personalized, risk-stratified, management guidelines. Innovations like self-collection of samples to increase screening access, innovative triage methods to optimize management of screen positives, and scalable and efficacious precancer treatment approaches will be key to further enhance the utility of prevention interventions.

Gastrointestinal cancers are a leading cause of cancer morbidity and mortality. Many gastrointestinal cancers develop from cancer precursor lesions, which are commonly found in individuals with hereditary cancer syndromes. Hereditary cancer syndromes have advanced our understanding of cancer development and progression and have facilitated the evaluation of cancer prevention and interception efforts. Common gastrointestinal hereditary cancer syndromes, including their organ-specific cancer risk and surveillance recommendations, are reviewed in this article. The management of common gastroesophageal, pancreatic, and colonic precursor lesions is also discussed, regardless of their genetic background. Further research is needed to advance chemoprevention and immunoprevention strategies.

This article explores the multifaceted landscape of oral cancer precursor syndromes. Hereditary disorders like dyskeratosis congenita and Fanconi anemia increase the risk of malignancy. Oral potentially malignant disorders, notably leukoplakia, are discussed as precursors influenced by genetic and immunologic facets. Molecular insights delve into genetic mutations, allelic imbalances, and immune modulation as key players in precancerous progression, suggesting potential therapeutic targets. The article navigates the controversial terrain of management strategies of leukoplakia, encompassing surgical resection, chemoprevention, and immune modulation, while emphasizing the ongoing challenges in developing effective, evidence-based preventive approaches.

In breast cancer (BC) pathogenesis models, normal cells acquire somatic mutations and there is a stepwise progression from high-risk lesions and ductal carcinoma in situ to invasive cancer. The precancer biology of mammary tissue warrants better characterization to understand how different BC subtypes emerge. Primary methods for BC prevention or risk reduction include lifestyle changes, surgery, and chemoprevention. Surgical intervention for BC prevention involves risk-reducing prophylactic mastectomy, typically performed either synchronously with the treatment of a primary tumor or as a bilateral procedure in high-risk women. Chemoprevention with endocrine therapy carries adherence-limiting toxicity.

Skin cancers, including melanoma and keratinocyte carcinomas, are responsible for increasing health care burden internationally. Risk stratification and early detection are paramount for prevention and less risky treatment to overall improve patient outcomes and disease morbidity. Here, the authors discuss the key concepts leading to skin cancer initiation and progression. The authors also outline precursor and progression models for melanoma and keratinocyte carcinomas, including discussion of genetic alterations associated with the various stages of progression. Finally, the authors discuss the significance of immunoediting and the drivers behind increased risk of cutaneous malignancy in the state of immune dysregulation.

Cancer continues to be one the leading causes of death worldwide, primarily due to the late detection of the disease. Cancers detected at early stages may enable more effective intervention of the disease. However, most cancers lack well-established screening procedures except for cancers with an established early asymptomatic phase and clinically validated screening tests. There is a critical need to identify and develop assays/tools in conjunction with imaging approaches for precise screening and detection of the aggressive disease at an early stage. New developments in molecular cancer screening and early detection include germline testing, synthetic biomarkers, and liquid biopsy approaches.

HEMATOLOGY/ONCOLOGY
CLINICS OF NORTH AMERICA

THE CLINICS ARE AVAILABLE ONLINE!
Access your subscription at:
www.theclinics.com

Preface

Early Cancer Detection in Focus

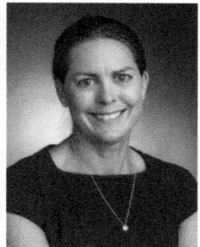

Elizabeth K. O'Donnell, MD
Editor

Early detection is a critical frontier in the ongoing battle against cancer. Tremendous progress has been made in the development of therapeutics for the treatment of cancer, which have led to significant improvements in disease survival. However, despite these advances, cure remains elusive for most advanced cancers. Improvements in diagnostic technologies, including liquid biopsy and advanced imaging, have created the opportunity to detect cancers at earlier stages. Multidisciplinary approaches that integrate expertise from diverse fields, such as oncology, genomics, imaging, bioinformatics, and artificial intelligence, are key to developing and validating innovative detection methods. In addition, investment in infrastructure, funding, and regulatory frameworks that support research and development in this area is crucial to translating scientific discoveries into clinical practice and ultimately improving patient outcomes. Public awareness and education also play a vital role in early cancer detection efforts. By promoting cancer screening programs, expanding access by reducing barriers, encouraging lifestyle modifications to reduce cancer risk, and empowering individuals to recognize early warning signs and seek medical attention promptly, we can further enhance the impact of research initiatives with the goal of saving lives. To move the needle on curing cancer, we must shift from a reactive to a proactive approach that encourages collaboration between researchers, clinicians, industry partners, and policymakers to accelerate progress in early cancer detection and cancer prevention.

In the special issue, we explore recent developments in cancer precursor conditions and their early detection. We begin with a discussion of the benefits and harms of early detection and interception of cancer by Dr Parmigiani. We then learn about the significant work that has been done in plasma cell precursors, including a review of clinical trials evaluating the treatment of precursor disease to prevent the development of symptomatic multiple myeloma by Drs O'Donnell, Borden, and Ghobrial. Drs Chang, Potter, Yang, and Sequist provide an update on lung nodule screening recommendations and novel screening techniques. Dr Sahasrabuddhe provides a state-of-the-art

Hematol Oncol Clin N Am 38 (2024) xi–xii
https://doi.org/10.1016/j.hoc.2024.04.006
0889-8588/24/© 2024 Published by Elsevier Inc.

hemonc.theclinics.com

review of cervical cancer precursors and prevention. We learn about gastrointestinal precursors conditions through the lens of hereditary predisposition syndromes from Dr Maoz, Rodrigues, Yurgelun, and Syngal. Drs Villa, William, and Hanna review hereditary predispositions to oral cancer and discuss oral potentially malignant disorders with a review of the therapeutic strategies. Ductal carcinoma in situ (DCIS) has probably been the most heavily studied to date. Drs Bychkovsky, Myers, Warren, De Placido, and Parsons discuss the disease biology of DCIS and primary and secondary prevention strategies. Drs Taylor, Nelson, and Dimitriou provide a comprehensive review of the landscape of cutaneous precursor conditions from genomics to early diagnosis. Finally, Drs Kohaar, Hodges, and Srivastava dive into the evolving science of blood biomarkers and liquid biopsy.

The significance of research into the early detection, and potentially the early interception of cancers, cannot be overstated, as it holds the promise of transforming cancer care by improving patient outcomes, reducing mortality rates, and easing the burden on health care systems worldwide. The goal of this issue is to bring into focus the importance of early detection and encourage research and discovery in this area.

DISCLOSURE

Research Funding: Regeneron; Advisory Board/Honoraria: Janssen, BMS, Sanofi, Pfizer, Exact Sciences, Grail; Consulting—Takeda; Steering Committee: Natera, Legend Pharmaceuticals.

Elizabeth K. O'Donnell, MD
Department of Medical Oncology
Dana-Farber Cancer Institute
Boston, MA 02215, USA

Harvard Medical School
Boston, MA 02215, USA

E-mail address:
elizabeth_odonnell@dfci.harvard.edu

Benefits and Harms of Interception and Early Detection of Cancer

Giovanni Parmigiani, PhD[a,b],*

KEYWORDS

- Cancer early detection • Screening • Interception • Risk–benefit analysis

KEY POINTS

- Screening for early detection and interception of cancer is characterized by 2 elements: *proactive search* for cancer and *proactive disruption* of cancer evolution.
- Benefits and harms vary widely depending on cancer types, screening modalities, target populations, treatments available for interception, and health care delivery approaches following diagnosis.
- Mapping benefits and harms requires comprehensive consideration of a life span and is best implemented via quantitative decision models.

INTRODUCTION

"Interception of cancer" has been defined as the "disruption of the oncogenic process during the precursor or pre-cancer state".[1] Interception typically involves active steps to identifying ongoing conditions that may favor the onset of carcinogenesis, and halting or reversing carcinogenesis at early stages, using pharmacologic approaches.[2] Intervention strategies may, for example, control mechanisms of early cancer development or boost immunity.[3]

"Early detection of cancer" has been defined as "the diagnosis and removal of cancer before there are metastases, and in the case of a pre-malignant lesion, before it becomes malignant." (Berlin, as cited by Miller[4]). Early detection may result from symptoms prompting medical care; from incidental findings during care administered for other reasons; or from screening, understood as a proactive effort to detect cancer early.[4] Early detection can improve options for an effective treatment and has been a central piece of cancer control practice for many years.[5,6] As we write, technological advances in early detection technologies are happening at a fast pace in most cancers via several modalities.[7–10]

[a] Department of Data Science, Dana Farber Cancer Institute; [b] Department of Biostatistics, Harvard T.H. Chan School of Public Health
* 450 Brookline Avenue, Boston, MA 02215.
E-mail address: gp@ds.dfci.harvard.edu

Hematol Oncol Clin N Am 38 (2024) 731–741
https://doi.org/10.1016/j.hoc.2024.04.003
0889-8588/24/© 2024 Elsevier Inc. All rights reserved.

There is some overlap in these definitions, but in general, cancer interception is synergistic and complementary to early detection and can take place independently when justified by a sufficiently high risk of developing cancer.[11]

The foundation for both approaches is in 2 elements: *proactive search* for cancer driver conditions or cancer itself and *proactive disruption* of cancer evolution. In interception, the search is most often based on risk stratification, possibly using molecular assays. The disruption may use bespoke treatments. In screening for early detection, the emphasis is on the search, and typically the disruption involves surgery or other treatments already available for early-stage cancers. Potential benefits of early detection and interception are compelling and have motivated both public health and clinical efforts. However, both early detection and interception strategies also have potential negative consequences.[12–14] Most of the benefits and risks of both approaches can be mapped back to the 2 fundamental elements of search and disruption.

When entirely successful, both screening and interception can avert the occurrence of cancer altogether. At the opposite extreme, screening for early detection can lead to imparting cancer treatment on individuals who would not otherwise have experienced cancer care. Similarly, interception strategies may treat individuals who would not have experienced cancer even if untreated. Generally, benefits and harms are more nuanced and multifaceted and exist for individuals, health systems, and society at large. **Table 1** summarizes the potential benefits and harms as relevant for an individual. Potential benefits include increases in length and quality of life, as well as decreases in morbidity and cost of treatment. Potential harms include overdiagnosis, overtreatment, as well as adverse effects and costs associated with the screening and interception activities themselves.

Investigating, quantifying, and communicating benefits and harms of interception and early detection are essential for effective and equitable cancer control. Recently, Castle and coauthors[14] have proposed the "Equal care for equal risk principle," which posits the risk/benefit trade-off as the organizing principle for implementing and evaluating cancer control interventions.

The benefits and harms of both screening and interception strategies will vary widely depending on the target populations, the types of cancer, the detection and interception modalities, and the delivery approaches of health care after diagnosis. Furthermore, the benefits and harms of both screening and interception strategies will play out over the course of many years and may affect health outcomes throughout the course of a lifetime. This article attempts to identify common elements that can inform the evaluation of early detection strategies in many of these scenarios.

MAPPING BENEFITS AND HARMS
Health States

A typical cancer evolves through stages whose negative manifestations are delayed compared to the underlying changes at the cellular level.[17] This delay can create a window of opportunity for early detection and interception. Also, many cancers may evolve through, or in association with, premalignant conditions.

Fig. 1 summarizes the essential elements of a lifetime history, as relevant for understanding and quantifying the benefits and harms of early detection and interception activities. These essential elements are represented as "health states" and as connections between health states that represent possible changes, or "transitions." **Fig. 1** can be interpreted as describing either an individual or a cohort. Here, I focus on the interpretation at the individual level. One can think of the graphs as subway maps, to be traversed only from left to right, via a single path, beginning with "no

Table 1
Categories (left) and examples (right) of benefits and harms of proactive searching and proactively disrupting cancer, for a single individual[a]

Potential benefits of proactive search	
Diagnosis at more favorable Stage	Diagnosis prior to the development of metastases
More accurate risk	Risk assessment following discovery of clonal hematopoiesis of indeterminate potential (CHIP)[15]
Potential benefits of proactive disruption	
Avoidance of malignancy	Curative resection of a localized mass that would have generated metastatic disease before becoming symptomatic (screening) or pharmacological control of the progression of a premalignancy (interception)
More effective treatment	Administration of a radiation treatment that is more effective in earlier than later stages
Less intensive treatment	Localized treatment as compared to a combination of localized and systemic treatments
Less costly treatment	Avoidance of treatment needed for disease in the late stage of the disease or resistant to therapy
Longer life	Results of the more effective treatment
Better quality of life	Results of the less intensive treatment
Potential harms of proactive search	
Overdiagnosis cancer diagnosis for a condition that would not have caused symptoms or harm during a patient's lifetime if not detected by screening[16]	
Adverse effects of screening	Complications arising from invasive procedures such as procedure endoscopy
Potential harms of proactive disruption	
Overtreatment	Treatment for a condition that would not have harmed the individual
Adverse effects of interception treatment	Side effects of pharmacological treatment
Worse quality of life	Psychological harm experienced after a diagnosis

[a] Categories are related and in part overlapping. Most apply to both screening for early detection and cancer interception.

cancer" and terminating with either "cancer-related death" or "death unrelated to cancer." Rectangles are stations. Travelers stay in a station until they transition to another to the right. The travel time here is zero, as in this representation an individual is always in one and only one health state.

The color scheme in **Fig. 1** is important. Black states are not directly observable and depict the underlying evolution of the cancer(s). Green health states are observable in the absence of screening, for example, when symptoms occur. Three red health states only exist in the presence of screening: detection of a precancer condition before it becomes symptomatic, detection of a malignant condition before it becomes symptomatic, and treatment of a condition detected as a result of screening. In the subway map analogy, black states are underground stations, while green and red states are on the surface. Comparing the top map (no interventions) with the bottom, interception and early detection strategies modify the map in many ways, such as adding new surface stations, adding new connections, and changing the frequency of trains on various connections.

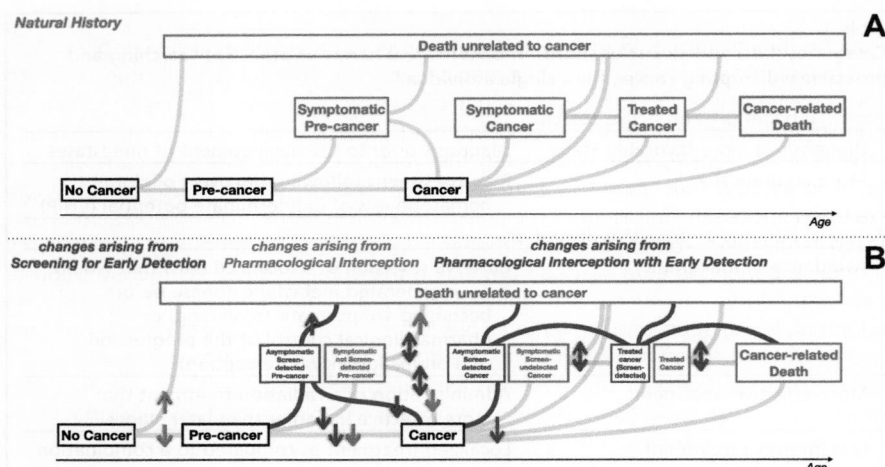

Fig. 1. Health states and transitions. Panels A and B represent the history of a cancer of interest, in the absence (presence) of screening for interception and early detection. Rectangles represent health states. Black states are not directly observable and depict the underlying evolution of the cancer. Green states are observable in the absence of screening, for example, as a result of symptoms. Red states only exist in the presence of a screening strategy. Connections between states represent transitions. These may occur at any age. Transition will occur from left to right. Gray transitions exist in the absence of screening, while red transitions are made possible by screening. Arrows represent changes in transition probabilities when comparing panel A to panel B, to show the likely effects of interventions.

The cancer type, the early detection and interception modalities, the screening implementation details, and the individual's risk factors for cancers and other diseases are all left unspecified. This is to highlight aspects common to most scenarios. One can also interpret the "cancer" state as a collection of malignancies for which a single detection or interception modality applies, as in multicancer early detection.[10]

For a given type of cancer, the definition of health states depends on the cultural, social, and health care context. Variation in these factors can substantially affect benefits and harms. For example, Koo and colleagues[18] note that "Psychological, social, and cultural factors influence the timeliness of help-seeking for symptoms. Individual and group level (eg, family or social network) barriers include cancer fear and stigma, poor health literacy, lack of trust in health care providers, and low expectations or perceptions regarding health care access or quality. Such barriers have been associated with demonstrably longer intervals to help seeking for possible cancer symptoms and advanced stage at diagnosis among those diagnosed with cancer."

CHIP[19,20] is a nonmalignant state characterized by mutation and clonal expansion of blood cells. Individuals with CHIP are at an increased risk of developing leukemia and other hematologic malignancies, as well as other diseases. Using CHIP as an example of precancer, an individual may enter the "precancer" health state at the time CHIP develops, and subsequently enter the "asymptomatic screen-detected precancer" health state when a blood test, taken while they were asymptomatic, reveals the condition. They may then remain in this state (whether treated or simply under surveillance) until they develop cancer, in which case they would move down to the black "cancer" health state until detected, or until they die at the end of a cancer-free life, in which case they move up to the "death unrelated to cancer" state.

Importantly, screening also changes the nature and clinical implications of the green states associated with symptomatic detection: "symptomatic not screen-detected precancer" and "symptomatic not screen-detected cancer" differ from their natural history counterparts. For example, in a regular screening program, cancer detected as a result of symptoms needs to have eluded previous early detection attempts, for example, by rapid growth.

The benefits and harms of detecting an asymptomatic premalignancy depend on whether the condition would itself have progressed to become a malignancy, a fact that is generally not knowable with certainty at the time of detection. If the premalignant condition can be removed or its evolution can be completely disrupted, this has the potential to completely avert a cancer, as is the case for polyps removed during colonoscopy screening.[21] Alternatively, early detection can support more targeted or more frequent screening approaches to facilitate the early detection of a later malignancy arising from or in association with the discovered premalignancy. In **Fig. 1**, this scenario is captured by a transition from "asymptomatic screen-detected precancer" to "cancer," followed by a transition from "cancer" to "asymptomatic screen-detected cancer." Additionally, screen-detection of premalignancies can be useful more broadly as a marker of risk, as is the case with CHIP. On the other hand, for premalignancies that would not eventually progress to malignant states, surgical removal and interception treatment are unnecessary procedures.

The benefits of detecting an asymptomatic malignancy depend on whether early detection leads to more effective treatment strategies. For example, the malignancy may be surgically curable when detected. This is a benefit of screening for an individual whenever the same malignancy would have progressed to the stage of not being surgically curable before becoming symptomatic—again a fact that is not generally knowable with certainty at the time of detection. Additionally, early detection can support more effective, though not fully curative, treatment. For example, gastrointestinal stromal tumors (GISTs) respond to tyrosine kinase inhibitors such as imatinib, but often develop drug resistance. Cells with mutations that confer resistance to imatinib are predicted to be present as subclones of a GIST at time of treatment, with probability that increases as a function of tumor size.[22] In this case, early detection can either decrease the chance that resistant subclones exist or prolong the time needed for the subclone to cause resistance.

On the other hand, screening carries the potential for overdiagnosis. For example, Draisma and colleagues[23] estimate the fraction of prostate cancers overdiagnosed by prostate specific antigen (PSA) screening using data from the European Randomized Study of Screening for Prostate Cancer, and 3 different modeling methods, and report estimates ranging from 23% to 42% of all cancers detected by screening. Overdiagnosis may lead to overtreatment; that is, administering treatments involving significant burden and side effects to individuals whose cancers would not actually need treatment.

Transitions

Fig. 1 also depicts possible transitions between states. Any individual will follow a single path along this network, from left to right, as they age. Gray transitions exist in the absence of screening, whereas red transitions are made possible by screening and are not present in the natural history scenario. The chance of making each of the outgoing transitions for someone in a given health state at a given age is called transition probability. Transition probabilities drive the balance of benefits and harms that underpins the evaluation of screening and interception strategies. Transition probabilities will depend on the age, the type or types of precancer/cancer, and specific risk factors of the individual depicted, such as the presence of cancer driver conditions. The time already spent in a state, in addition to age, will also affect transition probabilities. Transitions to and from states enabled by screening will depend on the sensitivity of the screening modality, its specificity, and other characteristics. Transition probabilities involving treatments will additionally reflect the treatment efficacy given the prior history.

Both interception and early detection intervention will affect the magnitude of transition probabilities. **Fig. 1** attempts to depict the probable direction of these changes, compared to natural history, using arrows. The direction of the arrow is up (down) if the transition probability is higher (lower) in panel B than in its counterpart in panel A. Some arrows point in both directions, to indicate that the change may go in either direction depending on the specific disease, intervention, and population considered. Colors are used to differentiate interception modalities. For example, red arrows refer to screening. Red arrows are not included for red transitions, as those do not exist in the natural history shown in panel A.

Screening for early detection will typically decrease the chance that an individual with a precancer condition will transition directly to cancer, as it creates a novel indirect path. It is, however, possible that overall the chances of transitioning from "precancer" to "cancer" remain unchanged when one considers all possible paths between these 2 states, in which case, the screening strategy is not effective in averting cancer onset. Similar considerations apply to transition out of the occult "cancer" state. Additionally, by affecting transition probabilities at early ages, screening can delay the onset of cancer or delay deaths related to cancer. Transition out of the "symptomatic not screen-detected precancer" and "symptomatic not screen-detected cancer" may be affected in either direction, depending on the nature of the premalignancies and malignancies that evade the screening modality considered. This is indicated by 2-pointed arrows.

Moving to interception, treatment of healthy individuals with an efficacious approach would reduce transition probabilities to precancer and cancer, and consequently increase the transition probabilities associated with a cancer-free life. Additional synergy may occur when combining early detection of premalignancies and interception, as interception may reduce the chance of developing a malignancy after detection of a premalignancy and conversely increase the chance of a cancer-free life (dark blue arrows in **Fig. 1**). Generally, transitions to "death unrelated to cancer" are indicative of a benefit from screening, except in the rare case of mortality attributable to the screening test itself.[24]

FACTORS AFFECTING THE EXTENT OF BENEFITS AND HARMS

The complex web of possibilities shown in **Fig. 1** highlights the challenges of comprehensively assessing the benefits and harms of screening for early detection and interception. Several factors need to be considered.

Cancer Type(s)

Various characteristics of a cancer's natural history can make it more likely for screening and interception to be beneficial. A slower progression through presymptomatic stages offers a longer window of opportunity for early detection and interception treatment. The existence of premalignant conditions that more frequently progress to malignancy, as in cervical or colon cancer, provides a rationale for surgical options following early detection. Cancers that are typically detected at a late stage, such as ovarian or pancreatic cancer, stand to offer greater benefit compared to cancers that often become symptomatic early enough for the treatment to be highly effective in the absence of a proactive search.

Early Detection Modalities

Overall specificity and sensitivity for detecting precancer will impact the risk–benefit balance of an early detection strategy. Generally, tests with low specificity will have greater risk of overdiagnosis. Tests with low sensitivity have a greater chance of missing early-stage disease. Populations screened with a low-sensitivity test would suffer the costs and potential dangers of the procedure with limited benefits. It is also important to understand the differences between premalignancies and malignancies that are detectable by a given screening modality, compared to those that are less easily detectable. For example, methods that detect tumor DNA in the blood or stool by searching for a prespecified set of DNA alterations may identify a set of cancer that is distinct at a molecular level from the set that is missed. This can be either positive or negative. For example, if early detection is followed by a targeted interception strategy that is likely to be effective in the favored subtype, the bias results in a useful synergy. On the contrary, if the test preferentially identifies indolent precancer or cancers that are less likely to ever become symptomatic, the bias results in higher rate of overdiagnosis compared to an unbiased detection. Depending on the modality, screening tests and follow-up diagnostic procedures carry intrinsic risks including complications, physical harm, radiation exposure, and other potential harms.

Disruption Modalities

Critical to the utility of early detection are the options available for interception and treatment following detection. If preinvasive or early-stage cancers cannot be cured or controlled with existing treatments, then early detection provides limited benefit. Regulatory evaluations of medical tests, for example the Centers for Medicare & Medicaid Services' determinations about coverage, pay close attention to clinical utility, that is a test's ability to have a positive impact on clinically meaningful health outcomes.[25] When combining search and interception, there are at least 2 important pathways to clinical utility: the first is the earlier administration of the same treatment that would have been given in the absence of a search, when this achieves greater effectiveness and the second is the ability to administer a better treatment regimen, either more efficacious or less onerous or both.

Target Population

Identifying the appropriate subgroup of individuals for specific interception or early detection efforts is critical to success. Using risk factors to focus screening toward higher risk groups can substantially affect the balance of benefits and harms associated with both early detection and disruption of cancer. Risk-based strategies can be designed to target those most likely to benefit while excluding lower risk individuals unlikely to develop symptomatic cancer. Risk stratification can leverage cancer driver conditions, as captured for example, by genetic (eg, pathogenic germline variants in genes related to familial cancer syndromes), behavioral (eg, smoking), or occupational (eg, radiation exposure) factors, as well as history of relevant premalignant conditions. For example, the National Comprehensive Cancer Network provides guidelines for cancer screening, detection, prevention, and risk reduction. These guidelines offer recommendations for various types of cancer screening, including colorectal and lung cancer screening and screening following genetic/familial high-risk assessment.[26,27] Most are based on risk stratification.

Risk stratification of prevention, early detection, and interception activities fit within the general paradigm of precision medicine[28] and can be described as precision early detection or interception.[11]

Cost

The cost of cancer screening can vary widely depending on the type of screening test, health care provider, and health care system. Although increased screening carries initial costs, an important question is whether earlier diagnosis could reduce overall medical costs, after one balances screening costs, overdiagnosis, and overtreatment on the one hand, and reduced treatment costs from early detection on the other hand, as fewer patients may require intensive treatments for advanced disease. Brill,[29] among others, provides an overview of the issues. Cost is an important consideration for public health programs and individuals and is a critical factor in determining access. Efforts to provide free or low-cost cancer screenings, testing, and vaccinations are essential for individuals who may not have adequate health insurance coverage.

Patient Preferences

Both screening procedures and early detection events carry psychological risks that must be weighed against individual values, as they affect different individuals to a widely ranging degree.[29] Patient preferences also show significant variability in how quality of life is weighed against duration of life. Earlier detection and interception aim to both extend life and also extend the fraction of life spent without debilitating effects of advanced disease and the associated treatment(s).

DECISION MODELING

Quantifying the relative importance of these benefits and harms is conceptually and practically challenging. Large studies with long follow-up are needed to observe a sufficient number of relevant events. It is not rare for screening modalities to be surpassed by the time the evidence from well-designed studies with sufficient follow-up matures. Even in the best studies, occult cancer states are not observable in unscreened populations. Often, empirical evidence is limited and challenging to interpret.

Formal decision models provide a constructive framework for weighing the many factors affecting the benefits and harms of screening and interception.[30–34] In concept, decision models can start with a map such as that of **Fig. 1**, where the health states, transitions, and interventions are no longer generic but are made specific to the disease(s) and intervention(s). Investigators need to use epidemiologic and clinical evidence, as well as expert judgment, to assign precise quantitative values to the transition probabilities for the connections between states. These will depend on age and stages as well as risk factors including genetics, behavioral, and environmental and will also account for screening and interception via a logic that quantifies the effects shown as arrows in **Fig. 1**. Once implemented, a decision model can generate, via simulation, cohorts of individuals with the desired risk stratification and detection/interception strategy, to support both bedside and policy decision-making, by quantifying benefits and harms in a way that is tailored to the population and health system under consideration.

Wilson and Jungner[35] proposed a set of principles to assess whether screening is appropriate. As recently revised by an expert consensus process,[36] the principles require that the cancer type "should be an important health problem, with well-understood epidemiology and natural history, a detectable preclinical phase, and clearly defined target population for testing."[13] Decision models can provide a quantitative evaluation of all these elements and support their coherent evaluation. Decision models can be used to drive cost-effectiveness and cost-utility analyses[32,37] as well as more informal or visual summaries.[38]

A number of useful decision models for cancer screening have been developed as part of the United States of America (U.S.A.) National Cancer Institute (N.C.I.s) Cancer Intervention and Surveillance Modeling Network,[39] a collaborative network of investigators who use simulation modeling to evaluate cancer control interventions. Breast cancer provides a good example of the scope and impact of these activities.[40]

LIMITATIONS

Having provided a rough conceptual outline to understand the benefits and harms of cancer screening and cancer interception, individually or jointly, I would like to close by mentioning some important limitations. The ostensible complexity of **Fig. 1** notwithstanding, most of the limitations of what I discussed this far lie in its oversimplifications.

Most cancers evolve through multiple stages, here condensed into "precancer" and "cancer." These stages differ with regard to (1) the underlying biology, potentially affecting the relevance of interception strategies; (2) the ability of detection modality to identify their presence prior to symptoms; (3) the risk of progression; (4) the treatments available; and (5) the implication for a person quality of life while in the condition. Malignancies with multiple preclinical states, such as multiple myeloma,[41] are not well modeled by the simplified view in **Fig. 1**.

Fig. 1 only depicts interception strategies that are applied to individuals prior to their first diagnosis of a malignancy in the cancer type(s) of interest. A higher resolution in the enumeration of premalignant and malignant cases could bring to focus a broader definition of interception, wherein interventions are also considered when detecting cancer at early stages of evolution, and when intercepting second cancers.

Fig. 1 does not consider the possibility that interception strategies may enhance or interfere with concomitant early detection strategies. For example, pharmacologic treatment may facilitate the detection of circulating tumor-generated nucleic acids.

Multiple modalities of detection are rapidly becoming more common. For example, less specific, noninvasive tests may be paired with more invasive but more accurate tests to be administered in case of a positive finding. The comparison of 2 individual modalities with natural history and with the combined use of both modalities would require 4 panels in an expanded **Fig. 1**. Possibilities grow multiplicatively as modalities are added. Interception can be interleaved in many ways when multiple modalities are in play.

Hopefully, by highlighting elements that are common to early detection and interception, and by providing a rough map for identifying the associated benefits and harms, this article will facilitate the evaluation of approaches specific to individual cancers, modalities, and populations.

DISCLOSURE

G. Parmigiani is cofounder of Phaeno Biotechnologies, consultant for Delfi Diagnostics, and scientific collaborator of Ambry Genetics. We acknowledge the Lavine family for generous support.

REFERENCES

1. National Cancer Institute. Cancer prevention-interception targeted agent discovery program. 2024. Available at: https://prevention.cancer.gov/major-programs/cancer-prevention-interception-targeted-agent-discovery-program-cap-it.

2. Blackburn EH. Cancer interception. Cancer Prev Res 2011;4(6):787–92.

3. Haldar SD, Vilar E, Maitra A, et al. Worth a pound of cure? emerging strategies and challenges in cancer immunoprevention. Cancer Prev Res 2023;16:483–95.
4. Miller DG. Principles of early detection of cancer. Cancer 1981;47(S5):1142–5.
5. Schiffman JD, Fisher PG, Gibbs P. Early detection of cancer: past, present, and future. American Society of Clinical Oncology Educational Book 2015;(35):57–65.
6. Crosby D, Bhatia S, Brindle KM, et al. Early detection of cancer. Science 2022; 375(6586). eaay9040.
7. Mattox AK, Bettegowda C, Zhou S, et al. Applications of liquid biopsies for cancer. Sci Transl Med 2019;11(507):eaay1984.
8. Fitzgerald RC, Antoniou AC, Fruk L, et al. The future of early cancer detection. Nat Med 2022;28(4):666–77.
9. Raoof S, Lee RJ, Jajoo K, et al. Multicancer early detection technologies: a review informed by past cancer screening studies. Cancer Epidemiol Biomarkers Prev 2022;31(6):1139–45.
10. Guerra CE, Sharma PV, Castillo BS. Multi-cancer early detection: the new frontier in cancer early detection. Annu Rev Med 2024;75(1). null.
11. Rebbeck TR, Burns-White K, Chan AT, et al. Precision prevention and early detection of cancer: fundamental principles. Cancer Discov 2018. https://doi.org/10.1158/2159-8290.CD-17-1415.
12. Bretthauer M, Kalager M. Principles, effectiveness and caveats in screening for cancer. Br J Surg 2012;100(1):55–65.
13. Medina JE, Dracopoli NC, Bach PB, et al. Cell-free DNA approaches for cancer early detection and interception. Journal for immunotherapy of cancer 2023;11.
14. Castle PE, Faupel-Badger JM, Umar A, et al. A proposed framework and lexicon for cancer prevention. Cancer Discov 2024;14:594–9.
15. Hoermann G. Clinical significance of clonal hematopoiesis of indeterminate potential in hematology and cardiovascular disease. Diagnostics 2022;12(7):1613.
16. Srivastava S, Koay EJ, Borowsky AD, et al. Cancer overdiagnosis: a biological challenge and clinical dilemma. Nat Rev Cancer 2019;19(6):349–58.
17. Stangis MM, Chen Z, Min J, et al. The hallmarks of precancer. Cancer Discov 2024;14(4):683–9.
18. Koo MM, Unger-Saldaña K, Mwaka AD, et al. Conceptual framework to guide early diagnosis programs for symptomatic cancer as part of global cancer control. JCO global oncology 2021;7:35–45.
19. Steensma DP, Bejar R, Jaiswal S, et al. Clonal hematopoiesis of indeterminate potential and its distinction from myelodysplastic syndromes. Blood 2015;126:9–16.
20. Weeks LD, Ebert BL. Causes and consequences of clonal hematopoiesis. Blood 1923;142:2235–46.
21. Kanth P, Inadomi JM. Screening and prevention of colorectal cancer. BMJ 2021;374.
22. Tomasetti C, Demetri G, Parmigiani G. Why tyrosine kinase inhibitor resistance is common in advanced gastrointestinal stromal tumors. F1000Research 2013;2(152).
23. Draisma G, Etzioni R, Tsodikov A, et al. Lead time and overdiagnosis in prostate-specific antigen screening: importance of methods and context. Journal of the National Cancer Institute 2009;101:374–83.
24. Kooyker AI, Toes-Zoutendijk E, Opstal-van Winden AWJ, et al. Colonoscopy-related mortality in a fecal immunochemical test-based colorectal cancer screening program. Clinical Gastroenterology Hepatol 2021;19:1418–25.
25. Hayes DF. Defining clinical utility of tumor biomarker tests: a clinician's viewpoint. J Clin Oncol 2021;39(3):238–48.

26. Daly MB, Pal T, Maxwell KN, et al. NCCN Guidelines® Insights: Genetic/Familial High-Risk Assessment: Breast, Ovarian, and Pancreatic, Version 2.2024: Featured Updates to the NCCN Guidelines. J Natl Compr Cancer Netw 2023;21(10):1000–10.
27. Ettinger DS, Wood DE, Aisner DL, et al. NCCN Guidelines® Insights: Non-Small Cell Lung Cancer, Version 2.2023: Featured Updates to the NCCN Guidelines. J Natl Compr Cancer Netw 2023;21(4):340–50.
28. Gillman MW, Hammond RA. Precision treatment and precision prevention: integrating "below and above the skin". JAMA Pediatr 2016;170:9–10.
29. Brill JV. Screening for cancer: the economic, medical, and psychosocial issues. Am J Manag Care 2020;26(Suppl 14):S300–6.
30. Zelen M, Feinleib M. On the theory of screening for chronic diseases. Biometrika 1969;56(3):601–14.
31. Eddy DM. Screening for cancer: theory analysis and design. SAddle River, NJ: Prentice-Hall; 1980.
32. Parmigiani G. Modeling in medical decision making: a Bayesian approach. Chichester: Wiley; 2002.
33. Gupta N, Verma R, Dhiman RK, et al. Cost-effectiveness analysis and decision modelling: a tutorial for clinicians. Journal of Clinical and Experimental Hepatology 2020;10(2):177–84.
34. Lange JM, Gogebakan KC, Gulati R, et al. Projecting the impact of multi-cancer early detection on late-stage incidence using multi-state disease modeling. Cancer Epidemiol Biomarkers Prev 2024. https://doi.org/10.1158/1055-9965.EPI-23-1470.
35. Wilson JM, Jungner YG. Principles and practice of mass screening for disease. Boletin de la Oficina Sanitaria Panamericana. Pan American Sanitary Bureau 1968;65:281–393.
36. Dobrow MJ, Hagens V, Chafe R, et al. Consolidated principles for screening based on a systematic review and consensus process. Canadian Medical Association journal 2018;190:E422–9.
37. Muennig P. Cost-effectiveness analyses in health: a practical approach. 2nd edition. Hoboken, NJ: Jossey-Bass; 2008.
38. Spiegelhalter D. Risk and uncertainty communication. Annual Review of Statistics and Its Application 2017;4(1):31–60.
39. National Cancer Institute. CISNET Modeling to guide public health research and priorities. 2024. Available at: https://cisnet.cancer.gov.
40. Alagoz O, Berry DA, de Koning HJ, et al. Introduction to the Cancer Intervention and Surveillance Modeling Network (CISNET) Breast Cancer Models. Med Decis Making 2018;38(1 suppl):3S–8S.
41. Heider M, Nickel K, Högner M, et al. Multiple myeloma: molecular pathogenesis and disease evolution. Oncol Res Treat 2021;44(12):672–81.

Early Detection of Precursor Diseases of Multiple Myeloma

Check for
updates

Elizabeth K. O'Donnell, MD[a,b,]*, Brittany A. Borden, MD[c],
Irene M. Ghobrial, MD[a,b]

KEYWORDS

- MGUS • Smoldering multiple myeloma • Precursor disease

KEY POINTS

- Precursor diseases of multiple myeloma, monoclonal gammopathy of uncertain significance and smoldering multiple myeloma, are prevalent and portend a risk of progression to multiple myeloma.
- There are ongoing efforts to best risk stratify, understand disease progression, and advance treatment possibilities in precursor diseases.
- Critical questions remain unanswered, including who should be screened for precursor diseases, which tools should be used, and who should be treated.

INTRODUCTION

Precursor diseases of multiple myeloma (MM), the most prevalent plasma cell dyscrasia, include monoclonal (M) gammopathy of undetermined significance (MGUS) and smoldering MM (SMM). It is well established that a percentage of affected individuals with each precursor disease will progress to MM, though which patients will progress is difficult to predict. Moreover, while treatment has been studied in precursor diseases, it is also not obvious which patients should be treated. Herein, precursor diseases are described, along with current risk stratification models and ongoing efforts to advance the understanding of disease progression and treatment.

DEFINING PRECURSOR DISEASES

MM arises from the malignant transformation of post-germinal center plasma cells. Essentially all cases of MM are preceded initially by MGUS, which is characterized by the presence of M protein.[1] M proteins are abnormal, clonal intact immunoglobulins

[a] Dana-Farber Cancer Institute, 450 Brookline Avenue, Boston, MA 02115, USA; [b] Harvard Medical School, 25 Shattuck Street, Boston, MA 02115, USA; [c] Brigham and Women's Hospital, 75 Francis Street, Boston, MA 02115, USA
* Corresponding author.
E-mail address: Elizabeth_odonnell@dfci.harvard.edu

Hematol Oncol Clin N Am 38 (2024) 743–753
https://doi.org/10.1016/j.hoc.2024.03.003
0889-8588/24/© 2024 Elsevier Inc. All rights reserved.

(Igs), predominantly IgG and IgA. The presence of an IgM M protein is typically associated with Waldenstrom macroglobulinemia, a lymphoplasmacytic lymphoma. By definition, MM is diagnosed by the presence of greater than or equal to 10% clonal plasma cells in the bone marrow (or biopsy-proven bony or extramedullary plasmacytoma) and the presence of a myeloma-defining event including evidence of end-organ damage including hypercalcemia, renal insufficiency, anemia, or bone lesions. In addition, greater than or equal to 60% clonal plasma cells in the bone marrow, a serum free light chain ratio greater than or equal to 100, or more than 1 focal lesion on MRI, all qualify as myeloma-defining events.[2]

MGUS is defined by the presence of M protein or abnormal free light chain ratio with less than 10% bone marrow plasma cells and the absence of myeloma-defining events.[2] Low-risk, intermediate-risk, and high-risk MGUS are described in the following sections. Importantly, the progression from low-risk MGUS to MM is approximated at 1% per year.[3] SMM is defined by the presence of M protein or abnormal free light chain ratio with 10% to 59% bone marrow plasma cells and the absence of myeloma-defining events.[4] As with MGUS, SMM can be further risk-stratified, as elaborated upon in the following sections. The progression from low-risk to high-risk SMM is approximated at 10% per year.[5] Notably, within the first 5 years following the diagnosis of SMM, 51% of affected individuals will convert to MM; moreover, an additional 27% will convert to MM in the subsequent 15 years.[6,7] Finally, an additional precursor disease called M gammopathy of indeterminate potential (MGIP) is defined by M protein less than 0.2 g/L on immunofixation; this precursor disease is predominantly represented by the IgM isotype.[8]

TOOLS FOR DIAGNOSIS

Initial diagnosis of precursor diseases is typically accomplished by serum protein electrophoresis (SPEP), urine protein electrophoresis (UPEP), serum free light chains, and immunofixation. SPEP detects the presence of M protein and enables assessment of the size of the M protein. However, the assay is not as sensitive when M proteins are small and the Ig heavy chain and light chain class cannot be determined.[9] UPEP is analogous to SPEP, detecting the presence of M protein in the urine. Immunofixation is more sensitive than SPEP and UPEP and is able to detect serum M protein greater than 0.2 g/dL and urine M protein greater than 0.04 g/dL.[10] Additionally, immunofixation allows for the determination of the isotype of the heavy chains and light chains, though it does not estimate the size of the M protein.[11] Moreover, serum free light chain assays measure concentrations of kappa and lambda free light chains, both clonal and normal free light chain not bound to the heavy chain.[12] Notably, new approaches, specifically mass spectrometry, can provide more precise detection in the diagnosis of MGUS as well as MGIP.[8] Importantly, the kappa to lambda ratio can be adjusted for kidney impairment[13] and, in fact, should also be adjusted in those of African descent based on abnormal light chain ratio at baseline.[8]

RISK STRATIFICATION OF PRECURSOR DISEASES

Risk stratification of precursor diseases can help inform prediction of progression to MM, in addition to treatment decisions. Stratification exists for both MGUS and SMM, with systems often separating precursor diseases into 3 groups—low-risk, intermediate-risk, and high-risk (**Table 1**). For MGUS, low-risk is defined as those patients with M protein less than or equal to 1.5 g/dL, IgG M protein, and a normal serum free light chain ratio. Intermediate-risk MGUS is defined as meeting 1 of the following 3 criteria: M protein greater than or equal to 1.5 g/dL, IgA or IgM M protein, or abnormal

Table 1			
Risk stratification of monoclonal gammopathy of uncertain significance			
Risk Category	Monoclonal Protein Quantity	Monoclonal Protein Isotype	Serum Free Light Chain Ratio
Low-risk	≤ 1.5 g/dL	IgM	Normal
Intermediate-risk[a]	≥ 1.5 g/dL	IgA or IgM	Abnormal
High-risk[b]	≥ 1.5 g/dL	Non-IgM	Abnormal

Abbreviations: Ig, immunoglobulin; MGUS, monoclonal gammopathy of uncertain significance.
[a] Having 1 of 3 criteria defines intermediate-risk MGUS.
[b] All 3 criteria required to be classified as high-risk MGUS.
From: Kyle RA, Durie BG, Rajkumar SV, et al. Monoclonal gammopathy of undetermined significance (MGUS) and smoldering (asymptomatic) multiple myeloma: IMWG consensus perspectives risk factors for progression and guidelines for monitoring and management. Leukemia. Jun 2010;24(6):1121-7. https://doi.org/10.1038/leu.2010.60

serum free light chain ratio. Finally, high-risk MGUS is defined as having M protein greater than or equal to 1.5 g/dL, IgA or IgM M protein, and an abnormal serum free light chain ratio.[14,15]

Three key risk models have been developed over the last 15 years for SMM, with new models currently being studied. The Spanish Programa para el Estudio de la Terapéutica en Hemopat´as Malignas (PETHEMA) risk model, published in 2007, takes into consideration aberrant plasma cells by immunophenotype plus immunoparesis for both MGUS and SMM patients. Patients with over 95% aberrant bone marrow plasma cells and immunoparesis had a 50% rate of progression at 2 years, while those with 1 of the 2 risk factors had a 35% rate of progression over the same period. Patients without either risk factor had a 5% risk of progression at 2 years.[16] The Mayo risk model, published in 2008, stratifies SMM patients according to the following risk factors: bone marrow plasma cells greater than or equal to 10%, serum M protein greater than or equal to 3 g/dL, and serum free light chain ratio either less than 0.125 or 8. Progression to MM at 2 years for 1, 2, or 3 risk factors were 12%, 27%, and 52%, respectively.[17] More recently, the 20/2/20 model was published in 2020. Three criteria are incorporated into this model: greater than 20% bone marrow plasma cells, greater than 2 g/dL M protein, and greater than 20 serum free light chain ratio. Those with 2 or 3 risk factors, deemed to be high-risk, had a risk of progression of 44.2% at 2 years, while those with 1 risk factor (intermediate risk) had a 17.9% risk of progression. Those with no risk factors had a 6.2% risk of progression at 2 years.[18]

Despite data supporting both statistical and clinical significance for risk stratification, the aforementioned models are not without their limitations. It is well known that precursor diseases exist as a spectrum; hence, MGUS and SMM indeed have overlap. However, most models consider MGUS and SMM as distinct entities, highlighting the need to capture intermediate states, such as MGUS-like SMM. Moreover, many of the aforementioned biomarkers evolve over time, and static models do not capture the dynamic nature of the disease course. It is also important to note that many of the models take into account bone marrow biopsy data; however, not all patients undergo initial or serial biopsies. Thus, a model without bone marrow biopsy as a significant criterion is desirable.

To combat such limitations, other models are being developed and additional criteria are being studied. For example, genomic data can be incorporated into the 20/2/20 model to increase predictive value. Specifically, high-risk fluorescence in situ hybridization data, including translocation (4;14), translocation (14;16), deletion 13q, and gain 1q, can further stratify patients, providing an additional predictor of progression.[18]

Additional genetic aberrations at the mutation level that could assist with risk stratification include mitogen-activated protein kinase pathway mutations and DNA repair mutations.[19] Moreover, circulating tumor cells (CTCs) have been shown to outperform bone marrow plasma cells in the assessment of SMM tumor burden.[20] Another predictive model, the PANGEA (Personalized Progression Prediction in Patients with MGUS or SMM) model, includes both MGUS and SMM patients, in addition to those with and without bone marrow biopsy data. Importantly, this model takes into account dynamic measures, such as hemoglobin decrease and creatinine, and has shown prediction improvement over the 20/2/20 model. Specifically, the PANGEA model that incorporates bone marrow biopsy data showed a 43% prediction improvement compared to the baseline 20/2/20 model and an 18% prediction improvement compared to the rolling 20/2/20 model. Similarly, the PANGEA model without bone marrow biopsy data showed a 30% and 22% prediction improvement compared to the baseline 20/2/20 and rolling 20/2/20 models, respectively. Notably, 58% of SMM patients who eventually progressed to MM were reclassified from a rolling 20/2/20 model intermediate-risk or low-risk category into the PANGEA high-risk category.[21] This perhaps highlights the importance of dynamic biomarkers in predictive models that can be reevaluated at multiple timepoints. Overall, the PANGEA model provides an avenue for assessing risk without bone marrow biopsy and importantly, can be applied to patients with MGUS or SMM. Further, new technology, such as single-cell sequencing, may be a promising avenue for diagnosis. Single-cell analysis can discriminate between CTCs and healthy cells, which can be used for MM prognostication and for assessing the risk of progression to MM.[22] It is possible that using such technology may alleviate the need for bone marrow biopsy. Further, the presence of CTCs can aid in obtaining patient-specific M protein sequences for more personalized approaches.[23]

SCREENING

Currently, screening guidelines for plasma cell disorders do not exist. Several important studies are currently being conducted to better understand the impact of screening in both broad populations and in focused, higher risk groups. The iStopMM (Iceland Screens, Treats, or Prevents Multiple Myeloma) study is a large, population-based screening study for MGUS that aims to identify candidates for early treatment in MM. Briefly, those in the study are screened with SPEP and serum free light chains; those identified as having MGUS are then randomized to 1 of 3 arms: no further workup, follow current guidelines, or more intensive follow-up.[24] Not only will this study provide data regarding which patients may be at higher risk of progression, but it will also illuminate the potential harms and benefits of early screening. Additionally, the PROMISE (Predicting Progression of Developing Myeloma in a High-Risk Screened Population; NCT03689595) study focuses on the development of a screening method for high-risk individuals to further elucidate factors that may contribute to precursor disease progression. Of note, while the study population of iStopMM is largely homogenous, the PROMISE study eligibility criteria include individuals with first-degree family members with blood cancers and/or African Americans. Taken together, these ongoing studies may provide a high degree of generalizability and help shed light on important, unanswered questions at this point: who to screen, who is more likely to progress to MM, and, ultimately, who to treat.

TREATMENT OF PRECURSOR DISEASES

Given the progression of precursor diseases, especially in high-risk patients, treatment for those affected deserves serious consideration. To that end, there have been several trials that have focused on treating SMM prior to progression to MM. There have been 2 phase 3 clinical trials that have focused on the use of lenalidomide. Mateos and colleagues[25–27] have studied lenalidomide plus dexamethasone in high-risk SMM. Notably, this treatment regimen showed sustained time-to-progression benefit, in addition to a sustained benefit in overall survival, compared to observation. Specifically, at a median follow-up time of 12.5 years, the median time to progression was 2.1 years in the observation arm and 9.5 years in the treatment arm. Moreover, the overall survival in the observation arm was 8.5 years and was not reached in the treatment arm. Lonial and colleagues[28] also conducted a phase 3 clinical trial comparing lenalidomide monotherapy to observation in patients with intermediate-risk or high-risk SMM. A significant progression-free survival (PFS) benefit was again seen, with a PFS rate of 91% in the treatment arm compared to 66% in the observation arm at 3 years. Taken together, these results suggest a possible role for lenalidomide, with or without dexamethasone, in those with intermediate-risk to high-risk SMM.

Several phase 2 clinical trials have also been conducted studying additional treatments in SMM (**Table 2**). The GEM-CESAR (A phase II multicenter study of carfilzomib, lenalidomide and dexamethasone (KRd) plus high-dose therapy with melphalan-200 and autologous stem cell transplantation, followed by consolidation with KRd, and maintenance with lenalidomide and dexamethasone in patients with high risk smoldering multiple myeloma (SMM) under 65 years) study treated those with high-risk SMM with carfilzomib, lenalidomide, dexamethasone, and stem cell transplant (SCT) with curative intent. At a median follow-up of 55 months, 94% of patients who received the aforementioned treatment remained progression-free.[29,30] Currently, it is uncertain whether this regimen is superior to lenalidomide and dexamethasone, as these regimens have not been directly compared. Carfilzomib, lenalidomide, and dexamethasone have also been studied in combination with daratumumab in the ASCENT (Aggressive Smoldering Curative Approach Evaluating Novel Therapies and Transplant) trial, which showed that 84% of patients became marrow measurable residual disease (MRD) negative, with a median time to MRD negativity of 6.6 months.[31] Daratumumab monotherapy has also been studied in the CENTAURUS (A Study to Evaluate

Table 2			
Phase 2 clinical trials in smoldering multiple myeloma			
Trial	**Patient Population**	**Treatment**	**Relevant Results**
GEM-CESAR[30]	High-risk SMM	Carfilzomib, lenalidomide, dexamethasone, stem cell transplant	94% progression-free at median follow-up of 65 mo.
ASCENT[31]	High-risk SMM	Carfilzomib, lenalidomide, dexamethasone, daratumumab	84% became marrow MRD negative. Median time to MRD negativity of 6.6 mo.
CENTAURUS[32]	High-risk or intermediate-risk SMM	Daratumumab	Median PFS $\geq$ 24 mo
B-PRISM[33]	High-risk SMM	Daratumumab, bortezomib, lenalidomide, dexamethasone	Overall response rate of 90% with 50% MRD negativity. Low rates of toxicity.

Abbreviations: MRD, measurable residual disease; PFS, progression-free survival; SMM, smoldering multiple myeloma.

3 Dose Schedules of Daratumumab in Participants with Smoldering Multiple Myeloma) trial, which showed median PFS greater than or equal to 24 months with 3 different dosing strategies.[32] Finally, the B-PRISM (Precision Intervention Smoldering Myeloma; NCT04775550) trial is underway, which is studying the combination of daratumumab, bortezomib, lenalidomide, and dexamethasone. Thus far, results have shown an overall response rate of 90%, with 50% MRD negativity. Importantly, no patients have discontinued therapy due to toxicity.[33]

In addition to the aforementioned trials, other considerations for treatment are being studied. Immunotherapy trials in relapsed and refractory MM, such as the CARTITUDE-1 (A Study of JNJ-68284528, a Chimeric Antigen Receptor T Cell (CAR-T) Therapy Directed Against B-Cell Maturation Antigen (BCMA) in Participants With Relapsed or Refractory Multiple Myeloma) and the MajesTEC-1 (A Study of Teclistamab in Participants With Relapsed or Refractory Multiple Myeloma) trials, have paved the way for the study of immunotherapy in SMM.[34,35] Current trials of ciltacabtagene autoleucel and teclistamab are underway in high-risk SMM. For example, the Immuno-PRISM (PRecision Intervention Smoldering Myeloma; NCT05469893) study focuses on the comparison between teclistamab and lenalidomide plus dexamethasone, and the CAR-PRISM (PRecision Intervention Smoldering Myeloma; NCT05767359) trial investigates the use of the Food and Drug Administration–approved chimeric antigen receptor T-cell ciltacabtagene autoleucel. Additionally, using genomic profiles for targeted therapy is another consideration, especially in those with translocation (11;14), for which venetoclax may provide benefit.[36] Further targeted combinations, such as elotuzumab-lenalidomide, ixazomib-lenalidomide, and isatuximab-lenalidomide, are being evaluated as well.[37,38] Importantly, the ITHACA (A Phase 3 Randomized, Open-label, Multicenter Study of Isatuximab (SAR650984) in Combination With Lenalidomide and Dexamethasone Versus Lenalidomide and Dexamethasone in Patients With High-risk Smoldering Multiple Myeloma; NCT04270409) trial is directly comparing isatuximab in combination with lenalidomide and dexamethasone to the standard therapy of lenalidomide and dexamethasone.[39] Further, the DETER-SMM (Daratumumab to Enhance Therapeutic Effectiveness of Revlimid in Smoldering Myeloma; NCT03937635) is a randomized phase III trial that compares daratumumab, lenalidomide, and dexamethasone to lenalidomide with dexamethasone in high-risk SMM.

Another component that must be considered in precursor diseases to prevent progression is lifestyle factors. Several studies have established obesity as a risk factor for the progression of MGUS to MM.[40,41] However, few studies have rigorously investigated dietary intervention to prevent disease progression. Both calorie restriction and intermittent fasting have been proposed as means to prevent further development of numerous cancers.[42] The PROFAST study (PROFAST Intervention in Precursor Multiple Myeloma; NCT05565638) is currently assessing whether prolonged nightly fasting impacts body composition and the risk of progression in overweight and obese patients with MGUS, SMM, and smoldering Waldenstrom macroglobulinemia. Moreover, studies have shown that metformin may play a role in preventing the development of MM in diabetic patients with MGUS and SMM.[43,44] A current randomized, placebo-controlled phase 2 study is assessing the effect of metformin on the progression to MM in those with high-risk MGUS and low-risk SMM.[45] Finally, studies have suggested that gut microbiome may influence the progression of precursor diseases to MM.[46] Plant-based diets and omega-3 fatty acid and curcumin supplements are being studied in the NUTRIVENTION (A Pilot Plant-Based Dietary Intervention in Overweight and Obese Patients With Monoclonal Gammopathy of Undetermined Significance (MGUS) and Smoldering Multiple Myeloma (SMM) - The Nutrition Prevention;

NCT04920084) study, as these interventions may impact butyrate, a substance with anti-inflammatory properties, in the gut microbiome.

While treating precursor diseases may prevent progression to MM, treatment is not without risks. It is well known that lenalidomide carries the risk of numerous side effects, including neutropenia, thrombocytopenia, increased risk of thromboembolic events, and various gastrointestinal side effects. Moreover, while the mechanism is not clearly established, lenalidomide use has been associated with an increased risk of secondary malignancies, such as acute myeloid leukemia, myelodysplastic syndromes, solid tumors, and non-melanoma skin cancers.[47] Reassuringly, in phase 3 clinical trials of lenalidomide and dexamethasone in high-risk SMM, only 1 lenalidomide-related death occurred due to a respiratory infection. Further, there was no significant difference in the risk of secondary malignancies between the treatment and observation arms. While the treatment regimen was overall well tolerated, the most frequent adverse events included infection, asthenia, neutropenia, and skin rash.[27] In other trials, grade 3 to 4 toxicities were seen in nearly half of those undergoing treatment. Specifically, such toxicities were seen in 44% of those on intensive daratumumab monotherapy in the CENTAURUS trial and 52% of those treated with daratumumab, carfilzomib, lenalidomide, and dexamethasone in the ASCENT trial.[31,32] Finally, in early studies of ixazomib, no patients discontinued treatment because of toxicity.[48] On the whole, it appears that treatment for high-risk SMM is well tolerated, though not without risk. Questions remain regarding how long to treat and whether SCT is eventually indicated for cure.

SUMMARY

To conclude, early detection of precursor diseases may ultimately prevent the development of MM. Critical questions remain to be answered; however, it is likely that we should be screening for precursor diseases, though guidelines regarding which patient populations should be screened, in addition to which tools should be used, do not yet exist. Sound data have been published regarding the benefit of treating precursor diseases, especially for those with high-risk SMM. Additional research should focus on whether treatment is warranted for low-risk and intermediate-risk SMM, in addition to MGUS. Finally, ongoing research is expanding the scope of possible treatment options for precursor diseases, from lenalidomide to multiple combination therapies to immunotherapy and beyond.

CLINICS CARE POINTS

- Precursor conditions of MM can progress to MM, though it can be challenging to predict which patients will progress.
- There are various tools for the diagnosis of precursor diseases, with additional tools currently being developed, though no screening guidelines currently exist.
- New and improved risk stratification models are currently being developed that incorporate additional factors, such as genomic data and dynamic measures of the disease.
- Various clinical trials are exploring possible treatment options for precursor diseases, though deciding on who to treat is not straightforward.

DISCLOSURE

O'Donnell: Steering Committee: Legend, Natera; Consulting/Honoraria: BMS, Janssen, Takeda, Sanofi, Exact, Grail, Pfizer; Travel: Grail, Sanofi. Ghobrial: Honoraria:

Celgene, Bristol-Myers Squibb, Takeda, Amgen, Janssen, Vor Biopharma Consulting or Advisory Role: Bristol-Myers Squibb, Novartis, Amgen, Takeda, Celgene, Cellectar, Sanofi, Janssen, Pfizer, Menarini Silicon Biosystems, Oncopeptides, The Binding Site, GlazoSmithKlein, AbbVie, Adaptive; 10xGenomics Travel, Accommodations, Expenses: Bristol Myers Squibb, Novartis, Celgene, Takeda, Janssen Oncology Spouse: William Savage, MD, PhD is the Chief Medical Officer at Disc Medicine and holds equity in the company Founder: PREDICTA Biosciences.

REFERENCES

1. Landgren O, Kyle RA, Pfeiffer RM, et al. Monoclonal gammopathy of undetermined significance (MGUS) consistently precedes multiple myeloma: a prospective study. Blood 2009;113(22):5412–7.
2. Rajkumar SV, Dimopoulos MA, Palumbo A, et al. International Myeloma Working Group updated criteria for the diagnosis of multiple myeloma. Lancet Oncol 2014;15(12):e538–48.
3. Kyle RA, Therneau TM, Rajkumar SV, et al. A long-term study of prognosis in monoclonal gammopathy of undetermined significance. N Engl J Med 2002; 346(8):564–9.
4. Lakshman A, Rajkumar SV, Buadi FK, et al. Risk stratification of smoldering multiple myeloma incorporating revised IMWG diagnostic criteria. Blood Cancer J 2018;8(6):59.
5. Rajkumar SV, Kumar S, Lonial S, et al. Smoldering multiple myeloma current treatment algorithms. Blood Cancer J 2022;12(9):129.
6. Kyle RA, Remstein ED, Therneau TM, et al. Clinical course and prognosis of smoldering (asymptomatic) multiple myeloma. N Engl J Med 2007;356(25):2582–90.
7. Greipp PR, San Miguel J, Durie BG, et al. International staging system for multiple myeloma. J Clin Oncol 2005;23(15):3412–20.
8. El-Khoury H, Lee DJ, Alberge JB, et al. Prevalence of monoclonal gammopathies and clinical outcomes in a high-risk US population screened by mass spectrometry: a multicentre cohort study. Lancet Haematol 2022. https://doi.org/10.1016/s2352-3026(22)00069-2.
9. Bradwell AR, Carr-Smith HD, Mead GP, et al. Highly sensitive, automated immunoassay for immunoglobulin free light chains in serum and urine. Clin Chem 2001; 47(4):673–80.
10. IMWG. Criteria for the classification of monoclonal gammopathies, multiple myeloma and related disorders: a report of the International Myeloma Working Group. Br J Haematol 2003;121(5):749–57.
11. Murray DL, Seningen JL, Dispenzieri A, et al. Laboratory persistence and clinical progression of small monoclonal abnormalities. Am J Clin Pathol 2012;138(4): 609–13.
12. Kyle RA, Gertz MA, Witzig TE, et al. Review of 1027 patients with newly diagnosed multiple myeloma. Mayo Clin Proc 2003;78(1):21–33.
13. Long TE, Indridason OS, Palsson R, et al. Defining new reference intervals for serum free light chains in individuals with chronic kidney disease: Results of the iStopMM study. Blood Cancer J 2022;12(9):133.
14. Rajkumar SV, Kyle RA, Therneau TM, et al. Serum free light chain ratio is an independent risk factor for progression in monoclonal gammopathy of undetermined significance. Blood 2005;106(3):812–7.
15. Kyle RA, Durie BG, Rajkumar SV, et al. Monoclonal gammopathy of undetermined significance (MGUS) and smoldering (asymptomatic) multiple myeloma: IMWG

consensus perspectives risk factors for progression and guidelines for monitoring and management. Leukemia 2010;24(6):1121–7.

16. Perez-Persona E, Vidriales MB, Mateo G, et al. New criteria to identify risk of progression in monoclonal gammopathy of uncertain significance and smoldering multiple myeloma based on multiparameter flow cytometry analysis of bone marrow plasma cells. Blood 2007;110(7):2586–92.

17. Dispenzieri A, Kyle RA, Katzmann JA, et al. Immunoglobulin free light chain ratio is an independent risk factor for progression of smoldering (asymptomatic) multiple myeloma. Blood 2008;111(2):785–9.

18. Mateos M-V, Kumar S, Dimopoulos MA, et al. International Myeloma Working Group risk stratification model for smoldering multiple myeloma (SMM). Blood Cancer J 2020;10(10).

19. Bustoros M, Sklavenitis-Pistofidis R, Park J, et al. Genomic Profiling of Smoldering Multiple Myeloma Identifies Patients at a High Risk of Disease Progression. J Clin Oncol 2020;38(21):2380–9.

20. Termini R, Zihala D, Terpos E, et al. Circulating Tumor and Immune Cells for Minimally Invasive Risk Stratification of Smoldering Multiple Myeloma. Clin Cancer Res 2022;28(21):4771–81.

21. Cowan A, Ferrari F, Freeman SS, et al. Personalised progression prediction in patients with monoclonal gammopathy of undetermined significance or smouldering multiple myeloma (PANGEA): a retrospective, multicohort study. Lancet Haematol 2023;10(3):e203–12.

22. Zavidij O, Haradhvala NJ, Mouhieddine TH, et al. Single-cell RNA sequencing reveals compromised immune microenvironment in precursor stages of multiple myeloma. Nature Cancer 2020;1(5):493–506.

23. Cascino P, Nevone A, Piscitelli M, et al. Single-molecule real-time sequencing of the M protein: Toward personalized medicine in monoclonal gammopathies. Am J Hematol 2022;97(11):E389–92.

24. Rögnvaldsson S, Love TJ, Thorsteinsdottir S, et al. Iceland screens, treats, or prevents multiple myeloma (iStopMM): a population-based screening study for monoclonal gammopathy of undetermined significance and randomized controlled trial of follow-up strategies. Blood Cancer J 2021;11(5):94.

25. Mateos MV, Hernandez MT, Giraldo P, et al. Lenalidomide plus dexamethasone for high-risk smoldering multiple myeloma. N Engl J Med 2013;369(5):438–47.

26. Mateos MV, Hernandez MT, Giraldo P, et al. Lenalidomide plus dexamethasone versus observation in patients with high-risk smouldering multiple myeloma (QuiRedex): long-term follow-up of a randomised, controlled, phase 3 trial. Lancet Oncol 2016;17(8):1127–36.

27. Mateos MV, Hernández MT, Salvador C, et al. Lenalidomide-dexamethasone versus observation in high-risk smoldering myeloma after 12 years of median follow-up time: A randomized, open-label study. Eur J Cancer 2022;174:243–50.

28. Lonial S, Jacobus S, Fonseca R, et al. Randomized Trial of Lenalidomide Versus Observation in Smoldering Multiple Myeloma. J Clin Oncol 2019. https://doi.org/10.1200/JCO.19.01740. JCO1901740.

29. Mateos M-V, Martínez-López J, Rodríguez-Otero P, et al. Curative Strategy (GEM-CESAR) for High-Risk Smoldering Myeloma (SMM): Post-Hoc Analysis of Sustained Undetectable Measurable Residual Disease (MRD). Blood 2022;140(Supplement 1):292–4.

30. Mateos M-V, Martinez Lopez J, Rodríguez-Otero P, et al. Curative Strategy (GEM-CESAR) for High-Risk Smoldering Myeloma (SMM): Carfilzomib, Lenalidomide

and Dexamethasone (KRd) As Induction Followed By HDT-ASCT, Consolidation with Krd and Maintenance with Rd. Blood 2021;138:1829.

31. Kumar SK, Alsina M, Laplant B, et al. Fixed Duration Therapy with Daratumumab, Carfilzomib, Lenalidomide and Dexamethasone for High Risk Smoldering Multiple Myeloma-Results of the Ascent Trial. Blood 2022;140(Supplement 1):1830–2.

32. Landgren CO, Chari A, Cohen YC, et al. Daratumumab monotherapy for patients with intermediate-risk or high-risk smoldering multiple myeloma: a randomized, open-label, multicenter, phase 2 study (CENTAURUS). Leukemia 2020. https://doi.org/10.1038/s41375-020-0718-z.

33. Nadeem O, Redd R, Mo CC, et al. B-PRISM (Precision Intervention Smoldering Myeloma): A phase II trial of combination of daratumumab, bortezomib, lenalidomide, and dexamethasone in high-risk smoldering multiple myeloma. J Clin Oncol 2022;40(16_suppl):8040.

34. Berdeja JG, Madduri D, Usmani SZ, et al. Ciltacabtagene autoleucel, a B-cell maturation antigen-directed chimeric antigen receptor T-cell therapy in patients with relapsed or refractory multiple myeloma (CARTITUDE-1): a phase 1b/2 open-label study. Lancet 2021;398(10297):314–24.

35. Moreau P, Garfall AL, van de Donk NWCJ, et al. Teclistamab in Relapsed or Refractory Multiple Myeloma. N Engl J Med 2022;387(6):495–505.

36. Avet-Loiseau H, Thiébaut-Millot R, Li X, et al. t(11;14) status is stable between diagnosis and relapse, and concordant between detection methodologies based on fluorescence in situ hybridization and next-generation sequencing in patients with multiple myeloma. Haematologica 2023. https://doi.org/10.3324/haematol.2023.284072.

37. Spencer A, Samoilova O, Chng WJ, et al. Impact of ixazomib-lenalidomide-dexamethasone therapy on overall survival in multiple myeloma patients: Analysis of the emerging-markets subgroup of the TOURMALINE-MM1 trial. EJHaem 2022;3(4):1241–51.

38. Dimopoulos MA, Richardson PG, Bahlis NJ, et al. Addition of elotuzumab to lenalidomide and dexamethasone for patients with newly diagnosed, transplantation ineligible multiple myeloma (ELOQUENT-1): an open-label, multicentre, randomised, phase 3 trial. Lancet Haematol 2022;9(6):e403–14.

39. Ghobrial I, Rodríguez-Otero P, Koh Y, et al. P-137: ITHACA, a randomized multicenter phase 3 study of Isatuximab in combination with Lenalidomide and Dexamethasone in high-risk smoldering Multiple Myeloma: safety run-in preliminary results. Clin Lymphoma, Myeloma & Leukemia 2021;21:S109–10.

40. Chang SH, Luo S, Thomas TS, et al. Obesity and the Transformation of Monoclonal Gammopathy of Undetermined Significance to Multiple Myeloma: A Population-Based Cohort Study. J National Cancer Institute 2017;109(5).

41. Thordardottir M, Lindqvist EK, Lund SH, et al. Dietary intake is associated with risk of multiple myeloma and its precursor disease. PLoS One 2018;13(11). e0206047.

42. Clifton KK, Ma CX, Fontana L, et al. Intermittent fasting in the prevention and treatment of cancer. CA Cancer J Clin 2021;71(6):527–46.

43. Chang SH, Luo S, O'Brian KK, et al. Association between metformin use and transformation of monoclonal gammopathy of undetermined significance to multiple myeloma in U.S. veterans with diabetes mellitus: a population-based cohort study. Lancet Haematol 2015;2(1):e30–6.

44. Boursi B, Mamtani R, Yang YX, et al. Impact of metformin on the progression of MGUS to multiple myeloma. Leuk Lymphoma 2017;58(5):1265–7.

45. Marinac CR, Redd RA, Prescott J, et al. A Randomized Placebo-Controlled Phase 2 Study of Metformin for the Prevention of Progression of Monoclonal Gammopathy of Undetermined Significance and Low Risk Smoldering Multiple Myeloma. Blood 2021/11/05/2021;138(Supplement 1):1659.
46. Antoine Pepeljugoski C, Morgan G, Braunstein M. Analysis of intestinal microbiome in multiple myeloma reveals progressive dysbiosis compared to MGUS and healthy individuals. Blood 2019;134(Supplement_1):3076.
47. Kotchetkov R, Masih-Khan E, Chu CM, et al. Secondary primary malignancies during the lenalidomide-dexamethasone regimen in relapsed/refractory multiple myeloma patients. Cancer Med 2017;6(1):3–11.
48. Nadeem O, Redd RA, Barth P, et al. A Phase I/II Study of Twice Weekly Ixazomib Plus Pomalidomide and Dexamethasone in Relapsed and Refractory Multiple Myeloma. Blood 2021;138(Supplement 1):1650.

Early Detection and Interception of Lung Cancer

Allison E.B. Chang, MD, PhD[a,b,c,1], Alexandra L. Potter, BS[d,1],
Chi-Fu Jeffrey Yang, MD[c,d], Lecia V. Sequist, MD, MPH[a,c,*]

KEYWORDS

- Lung cancer • Lung cancer screening • Cancer risk • Early detection • Disparities
- Artificial intelligence

KEY POINTS

- Lung cancer is the leading cause of cancer-related death, in large part because it tends to be diagnosed at an advanced stage, when cure is no longer possible.
- Lung cancer screening (LCS) with annual low-dose computed tomography (LDCT) is recommended for high-risk individuals with a significant smoking history, but uptake has been poor, with only approximately 5% of eligible people obtaining screening, and even fewer adhering to subsequent annual screening.
- Barriers to LCS implementation include: stigma related to lung cancer and smoking, lack of physician awareness, complexity of identifying eligible patients, limited access to LCS centers, and lack of insurance coverage.
- Many patients diagnosed with lung cancer would not have qualified for screening, indicating that the field must gain a better understanding of lung cancer risk factors besides simply age and tobacco exposure and should refine screening eligibility guidelines accordingly.
- A multipronged approach of both grassroots- and government-level activism is improving LCS awareness and uptake. Novel technologies have the potential to complement LDCT screening, or replace it altogether, which will undoubtedly improve clinicians' ability to risk stratify pulmonary nodules, detect early-stage lung cancers, and increase opportunities for LCS in communities that traditionally have had limited access to LDCT imaging.

INTRODUCTION

Recent advances in lung cancer treatment and waning smoking prevalence have led to dramatic improvements in 5-year survival rates, with a near doubling from the early 2000s, from approximately 15% to 25%.[1] But despite this progress, lung cancer

[a] Department of Medicine, Division of Hematology/Oncology, Massachusetts General Hospital, Boston, MA, USA; [b] Department of Hematology/Oncology, Dana Farber Cancer Institute, Boston, MA, USA; [c] Harvard Medical School, 25 Shattuck Street, Boston, MA 02115, USA; [d] Division of Thoracic Surgery, Department of Surgery, Massachusetts General Hospital, Boston, MA, USA
[1] Contributed equally.
* Corresponding author. Massachusetts General Hospital, 55 Fruit Street, Boston, MA 02114.
E-mail address: lvsequist@mgb.org

Hematol Oncol Clin N Am 38 (2024) 755–770
https://doi.org/10.1016/j.hoc.2024.03.004
0889-8588/24/© 2024 Elsevier Inc. All rights reserved.

causes approximately 130,000 deaths each year in the United States (US), remaining the leading cause of cancer-related mortality.[2] A major driver of lung cancer's lethality is the tendency to be diagnosed at an advanced stage. Nearly 50% of lung cancer patients are diagnosed when the cancer has spread to distant organs, and treatments for this group are usually not curative. Conversely, excellent outcomes can be achieved for stage I lung cancer, with 5-year survivals between 65% and 90%.[3] Several recent landmark trials have established new standards in perioperative therapy, incorporating both immunotherapy and targeted agents, which will likely lead to even higher cure rates for early-stage lung cancer in the coming years.[4–8] Surgical techniques are becoming more sophisticated and less invasive, which may also improve outcomes.[9,10] Moreover, stereotactic body radiotherapy has also provided patients with early-stage disease who are medically inoperable a greater chance at cure.[11]

Because of the vast differences in outcomes depending on stage at diagnosis, screening is critical to reduce lung cancer mortality by intercepting the disease at an earlier stage, when it has not yet caused symptoms. The data supporting lung cancer screening (LCS) will be reviewed herein, but despite endorsement by the United States Preventive Services Task Force (USPSTF) in 2013, routine LCS has been poorly adopted in the US, capturing less than 5% of eligible people nationally, and as little as 1% in some states.[12] By contrast, screening rates for breast and colorectal cancers in the US are 72% and 63%, respectively.[13] The reasons for poor uptake of LCS are likely multifactorial, because of a combination of stigma around lung cancer's relation to smoking, inadequate insurance coverage, proximity of patients to hospitals offering screening, physician awareness, and complexity in identifying eligible patients.[10,14] This article will describe the data supporting LCS, the obstacles to LCS implementation (focusing primarily on the US), and the promising opportunities that lie ahead.

THE HISTORY OF LUNG CANCER SCREENING

The search for effective LCS tests began in the early 1950s with observational and non-randomized studies focused on screening with chest radiograph (CXR), with or without sputum cytology.[15–19] However, none of these early studies showed a lung cancer mortality reduction, likely due to CXR's limited sensitivity. Then, the 1970s and 1980s saw a surge in lung cancer incidence, reflecting widespread smoking mid-century. This led to a renewed interest in LCS. The National Cancer Institute (NCI) sponsored 3 randomized trials designed to assess whether LCS programs could reduce lung cancer mortality: the Memorial Sloan-Kettering, Johns Hopkins, and Mayo Lung Projects. These trials were limited by their reliance on CXR and sputum cytology and had relatively small sample sizes. Once again, these trials found no significant difference in outcomes.[20–22] As a result, in 1996, the USPSTF recommended against LCS with CXR or sputum cytology. Finally, the Prostate, Lung, Colorectal, and Ovarian (PLCO) Cancer Screening trial sought to address the shortcomings in earlier trials, enrolling about 155,000 US participants between 1993 and 2001, randomized to either usual care (ie, no screening) or annual screening with CXR for up to 4 years.[23] The PLCO study confirmed the findings from the aforementioned studies, providing definitive evidence that screening via CXR does not reduce lung cancer mortality.

While the PLCO was ongoing, others pursued the possibility of LCS with low-dose computed tomography (LDCT), a new technology that boasted significantly improved sensitivity to detect small nodules through 3-dimensional imaging. The Early Action Lung Cancer Project was a single-arm prospective cohort study evaluating annual LCS using both CXR and LDCT in each subject. An analysis of the first 1000 participants found that screening with LDCT identified a greater number of lung cancers compared with screening with CXR, and 85% of cancers diagnosed were stage I.[24] These data provided strong support that LDCT was a more sensitive LCS modality than CXR, but the study's single arm nature prohibited evaluation of lung cancer mortality.

To evaluate whether LDCT-based screening could improve lung cancer mortality, a randomized trial was needed. The NCI sponsored the National Lung Screening Trial (NLST), a randomized controlled trial of high-risk participants, based on empirically selected age (55 years–74 years) and tobacco history (30 pack-year) cut-offs. Over 53,000 individuals were randomized to up to 3 years of annual screening with LDCT or CXR. In 2011, just 3 months before the PLCO findings were published, the NLST results were published demonstrating that screening with LDCT resulted in a 20% reduction in lung cancer mortality and 6% reduction in all-cause mortality compared with CXR.[25]

After the NLST, several smaller European randomized trials, including DANTE, DLCST, the MILD trial, and the NELSON trial, compared LDCT screening to either no screening or CXR-based screening.[26–30] The largest of these trials, NELSON, similarly found that LCS significantly reduced lung cancer mortality by 24% to 33%.[29] While the other trials were not powered to detect a reduction in lung cancer mortality, a meta-analysis indeed confirmed that screening with LDCT significantly reduced lung cancer mortality, providing further evidence supporting LCS.[31]

IMPLEMENTATION OF LOW-DOSE COMPUTED TOMOGRAPHY SCREENING IN THE UNITED STATES
2013 United States Preventive Services Task Force Recommendation

In December 2013, the USPSTF endorsed LCS for the first time, recommending annual LDCT for individuals aged 55 years to 80 years with at least a 30 pack-year smoking history who currently smoke or quit smoking within the past 15 years.[32] The Grade B recommendation from the USPSTF meant that most private health insurances would be mandated to cover LCS as a preventive service. When the Centers for Medicaid and Medicare Services (CMS) added LCS to their coverage list in 2015,[33] it was hoped that screening would be quickly taken up and widely utilized across the country, with an estimated 10.7 million screening scans projected within the Medicare population over 5 years.[34] However, this was not the case. Indeed, it was not until 2019 that the US reached 1 million patients screened for lung cancer.[35]

Development and Implementation of the Lung-RADS System

A major challenge in LCS implementation has been minimizing false positives while maintaining sensitivity. In the NLST, the size cut-off for considering a new (or growing) nodule to be suspicious was greater than 4 mm and management decisions were standardized based on the size of the nodule and changes in size and characteristics compared with prior examinations.[25] While this standardized approach was designed to minimize false positives, the 4 mm threshold led to a 26% false positive rate, which raised concerns about potential costs and harms of LCS programs.[36,37]

In response, the Lung CT Screening Reporting and Data System (Lung-RADS) was developed by the American College of Radiology to reduce the false positive rate, standardize LDCT reporting, and improve management of positive findings. Analogous to the Breast imaging-reporting and data system (BI-RADS) for reporting mammography, Lung-RADS categorizes screen-detected lung nodules based on size, morphology (eg, non-solid, part-solid, or solid), and changes over time. Follow-up recommendations were also based on the Lung-RADS category. Importantly, the size threshold for a suspicious solid or part-solid nodule detected on a baseline LDCT exam was increased to 6 mm under Lung-RADS. Pinsky and colleagues retrospectively applied the Lung-RADS criteria to LDCT examinations from the NLST and compared the performance of Lung-RADS with the criteria for nodule management used in NLST.[38] They found that Lung-RADS resulted in substantial reductions in false positive rates, from 26.6% to 12.8% for the baseline examination and from 21.8% to 5.3% for subsequent LDCT examinations. Importantly, Lung-RADS maintained good sensitivity at 84.9% for the baseline scan (compared with 93.5% by NLST criteria).

Determining When to Biopsy

One of the most complicated aspects of lung cancer early interception is determining how to manage screen-detected lung nodules and minimize unnecessary invasive procedures. A multitude of clinical guidelines have been developed for lung nodule assessment and management, taking into account variables such as age, sex, emphysema, family history of lung cancer, and nodule characteristics (size, number, location, attenuation, and spiculation) to estimate the risk of a given nodule being cancerous.[39–44] In order to optimally apply the guidelines to individual patients and determine management recommendations, establishment of multidisciplinary pulmonary nodule clinics has been touted by organizations such as the National Comprehensive Cancer Network. In a pulmonary nodule clinic, experts from different specialties (eg, pulmonology, thoracic surgery, medical oncology, radiation oncology, and imaging) review cases together and build consensus recommendations.[45–47] Dedicated nodule clinics may be able to improve adherence to follow-up recommendations and allow for optimal patient triage for both invasive procedures and empiric cancer treatments (such as radiation) among those who cannot tolerate invasive procedures.[48–50]

Lung nodule programs are also critical for monitoring cancer risk in individuals who are incidentally found to have lung nodules but who do not qualify for annual LCS. For example, in Baptist Health System's pulmonary nodule clinic, over 50% of patients diagnosed with lung cancer through the nodule clinic were ineligible for screening under USPSTF guidelines.[51] Importantly, the cumulative lung cancer diagnosis hazard of screening-age persons enrolled in the lung nodule program was significantly higher than that among LCS program participants, and those diagnosed through the lung nodule clinic were more likely to be Black, uninsured, or age-ineligible for enrollment into Medicare.[52]

Low Uptake and Adherence in Lung Cancer Screening

Despite improvements in insurance coverage and reporting systems, lung screening uptake in the US has been extraordinarily slow. Multiple factors likely contribute. Awareness of LCS is low; one study found that 84% of high-risk Americans were unfamiliar with the screening.[53] In addition, cost remains a barrier for many individuals, especially those with certain state Medicaid plans or no insurance. Not only is the LDCT scan itself expensive, but also the possibility of downstream costs looms – a positive scan could lead to additional imaging, biopsies, and even cancer treatment. This creates a major financial barrier that deters some high-risk individuals from getting screened.[54] Limited access to LCS centers also prevents high-risk individuals from getting screened, especially those living in rural locations or those with full-time jobs who are unable to take time off work.[54] One study found that in rural areas, 25% of screening-eligible individuals lived at least 40 miles away from the closest LCS center[55]; this distance can be insurmountable for individuals without transportation or who work inflexible jobs. Several studies have also reported that the inability to take time off work is a major barrier to LCS.[56]

The dearth of available LCS sites is not simply related to population density. Policy design choices also may have negatively affected screening uptake in the US. For example, health care sites must document several unique requirements to receive reimbursement for LDCTs through CMS, including shared decision making and participation in a national database. These complexities are not required for other cancer screening tests and may have hindered establishment of LCS programs, though robust data are lacking.[57-61]

Equally concerning as LCS low uptake is low adherence to annual screening. Specific screening programs previously reported adherence to LCS in the range of 40% to 65% in real world practice,[62-64] but shocking data from the US national database of LCS revealed that among 1 million people who underwent a baseline LDCT from 2015 to 2019, the adherence rate to annual screening was only 22.3%.[35] This low adherence is particularly concerning given that the full benefits of cancer screenings are greatest when eligible individuals participate over time.

TOBACCO USE, STIGMA, RACE, AND UPDATED LUNG CANCER SCREENING GUIDELINES

There is no scientific doubt that tobacco use is linked to some cases of lung cancer. But historically, the role of tobacco in lung cancer etiology may have been over-simplified – conceptualized as the one and only explanation for a lung cancer in anyone with a history of tobacco use. Modern advances in genomics and epidemiology have pointed to air pollution as a significant cause of lung cancer, and increasing proportions of patients with lung cancer are now identified to have both somatic and germline genetic lesions, which are independent from tobacco exposure.[65-71] The cleanest example that lung cancer can be completely unrelated to tobacco is the rapidly rising proportion of patients with lung cancer who have never used tobacco,[72-74] though most likely a portion of lung cancers in people with tobacco exposure have been misattributed to tobacco use when in fact, the cancers are biologically driven by other factors.

Ironically, the use of smoking history as a selection criterion for LCS presents several important barriers to screening uptake. First, cigarette smoking has been heavily stigmatized over the last several decades. The stigma associated with smoking, and the perception that individuals who smoke and get lung cancer have "self-inflicted" disease, have proven significant barriers to increasing LCS.[75,76] Second, the use of smoking history to determine screening eligibility makes identifying LCS candidates a challenging and elusive task. Other common cancer screenings, including breast, colorectal, and cervical cancer screening, are based primarily on age and are therefore much simpler for patients and providers to know who is eligible. In contrast, LCS eligibility criteria are far more complicated, including not only age requirements but also detailed smoking history requirements (ie, pack-years and years since quitting smoking). Presently, smoking history routinely collected in the Electronic Health Record (EHR) is often insufficient to determine screening eligibility (ie, does not include all necessary information to calculate pack-years or quit years). For example, in a study of medical directors from 258 Federally Qualified Health Centers (FQHC), only 13% reported that their FQHC collected sufficient tobacco use data to determine lung cancer screening eligibility.[77] Additionally, even when sufficient tobacco use data is collected to determine eligibility, these data have been shown to be inaccurate. Most notably, pack-year smoking history in the EHR is often underestimated, inaccurately classifying many high-risk individuals who are eligible for screening as ineligible.[78,79] The stigma against smoking undoubtedly contributes to this systematic underestimation of smoking history.

Eligibility criteria for the definitive trials studying LCS were derived for the successful recruitment and conduct of the trial, not necessarily because they are the optimal criteria for population-level screening programs. And yet, of course, evidence from such trials form the foundation supporting screening guidelines. Both the NLST and NELSON trials were predominantly comprised of white men (indeed, the NELSON cohort was only 16% female[29]), so initial USPSTF guidelines were likely best suited to identify high-risk white men. Indeed, myriad studies have shown that racial minorities and women develop lung cancer at a younger age and with less smoking exposure than white men, suggesting that the age and pack-year criteria used to select patients for LCS were systematically excluding women and minorities from screening.[80–85] In 2021, USPSTF made amendments to their guidelines for screening with a goal of decreasing these disparities.[86] The updated guidelines recommended annual LDCT for adults aged 50 years to 80 years who have at least a 20 pack-year smoking history and currently smoke or have quit within the past 15 years. While it remains to be seen if the 2021 update in criteria will improve disparities in practice, the findings from numerous (but not all) retrospective analyses examining this question suggest that it will fall notably short.[82,87–96] Still, in order for equity to be meaningful, the system must ensure broad uptake of LCS overall, an objective at which it continues to fail notably in 2022.[12]

One other key issue with LCS eligibility criteria is the years since quitting criterion. The NLST arbitrarily chose 15 years from the quit date as a cut-off for trial eligibility, and hence, guidelines have followed that template. However, historic and emerging research has failed to demonstrate an inflection point in the decline in lung cancer risk at 15 years; rather, risk seems to decline slowly and steadily over time without a clear inflection point.[97,98] These findings led to the American Cancer Society's recent recommendation in November 2023 to remove the years since quitting requirement from LCS eligibility criteria.[99] At this time it is unknown if this recommendation will be echoed by the USPSTF, but clearly, the momentum to make LCS more accessible is strong. In their own research, the authors have found quantifying tobacco exposure by smoking duration, rather than pack-years, may improve the selection of individuals for LCS and allow for more equitable screening criteria.[100]

Screening guidelines should continue to evolve to best capture individuals with a variety of risk factors, especially those outside tobacco. Other risk factors for non-smoking-related lung cancer include radon exposure, asbestos exposure, and other occupational exposures. For example, there is particular concern related to burn pit exposure in the military, which was prevalent during the Iraq War.[101,102] Underlying lung disease and family history of lung cancer also significantly increase lung cancer risk. Importantly, lung cancer risk increases with low socioeconomic status.[103] Future work must focus on better understanding non-smoking risk factors for developing lung cancer and incorporating these risks into screening guidelines.

REASONS FOR OPTIMISM

Despite the low uptake of LCS in the US, there have already been measurable beneficial effects from screening over the last decade. Several studies have shown that since LDCT screening was first recommended by the USPSTF in 2013, there has been a significant increase in the proportion of early-stage lung cancers diagnosed in the US.[104–107] Among individuals in the US aged 55 years to 80 years, the percentage of NSCLC cases diagnosed at stage I (as opposed to later stages) increased by nearly 4% per year from 2014 to 2018, while fewer patients were diagnosed with stage III or IV NSCLC.[104] Encouragingly, these data show that screening even a relatively small number of eligible patients result in a beneficial lung cancer stage shift at the population level. At the same time, these data highlight the tremendous potential for LDCT screening to increase lung cancer early detection and reduce lung cancer mortality if it were to be broadly implemented.

Activism

Creative and innovative efforts to increase awareness of and access to LCS have flourished over the last several years. Several institutions, including Roswell Park in New York, CHI Memorial in Tennessee, Atrium Health in North and South Carolina, and West Virginia Cancer Institute in West Virginia, have deployed mobile LCS units, which bring lung screening "to the people," circumventing the financial and logistical challenges of traveling to brick-and-mortar screening clinics. Preliminary data have been promising, showing that mobile LCS units can facilitate high throughput and can identify lung cancers at a rate comparable to or even higher than that reported in the NLST.[108,109] Importantly, the patient population screened by mobile screening units tends to represent a more underserved patient population when compared with the patient population screened at traditional LCS clinics.

Another important effort to increase lung screening awareness and access has been grassroots-based community outreach and advocacy. The American Lung Cancer Screening Initiative (ALCSI) is a 501c(3) non-profit focused on increasing LCS awareness and helping high-risk individuals access screening (note authors Potter and Yang are the President and Founder/Director of ALCSI, respectively). ALCSI has a team of over 700 student volunteers across the US, with 51 ALCSI chapters in college campuses across the nation. To date, ALCSI has held over 450 community events and has educated over 15,000 community members about the importance of LCS. ALCSI has also worked with local and state leaders, including mayors, governors, state representatives, and doctors to film over 90 public service announcements about LCS; through these public service announcements, community leaders encourage high-risk individuals to get screened for lung cancer.

On a national level, ALCSI has worked with US congress members and senators to draft and advocate for the first-ever US House and Senate resolutions recognizing the importance of the early detection of lung cancer through screening. Notably, every year since 2020, the US Senate has passed Senate Resolutions (S.Res.780, S.Res.462, S.Res.863, and S.Res.512) with unanimous consent, cementing their support for early lung cancer detection and opening the path for new legislation to expand LCS access. The Increasing Access to Lung Cancer Screening Act was recently introduced in the US House and Senate and aims to improve access to LCS by requiring all state Medicaid programs to cover LCS, expanding Medicaid coverage for tobacco cessation counseling and treatment without prior authorization, and appropriating funds to support the development of an LCS registry.

Several US states have taken initiative to promote broad LCS implementation in their state. In Kentucky, the Kentucky Lung Cancer Education Awareness Detection Survivorship Collaborative was launched in 2014 with a specific focus on promoting high-quality LCS implementation through primary care provider education and supporting the development and maintenance of high-quality screening programs. As a result, Kentucky has one of the highest LCS rates in the US. In New Jersey, ScreenNJ is a statewide program focused on increasing access to cancer screenings, including LCS, through eliminating barriers.

Emerging Technology

In the last few years, advances in artificial intelligence and genomic sequencing have led to an explosion of new technologies in cancer diagnostics and early detection.[110] Broadly speaking, these tools are based on sophisticated classifiers trained to recognize patterns among vast amounts of data. Such classifiers can recognize genomic bar codes (eg, patterns of DNA methylation) and extract information from images beyond what human radiologists can detect. This has been particularly exciting for LCS, where together, these new tools could help with identifying at-risk individuals, detecting nodules with exquisite sensitivity, and risk stratifying positive scans. Novel screening tools could serve as an adjunct to LDCT, or perhaps, circumvent the need for LDCT altogether, thereby promoting uptake and adherence through more accessible tests; for example, a blood draw or bedside breath test.[111–114]

Machine learning has significantly increased the information that can be gleaned from a radiology image. One benefit is that it can be used to improve sensitivity for detecting subtle abnormalities. This improves both detection and risk stratification of small pulmonary nodules.[115–121] Some nodule risk stratification algorithms have demonstrated improved sensitivity and specificity compared with Lung-RADS and are already commercially available, having gained approval by the US Food and Drug Administration. Using machine learning to augment scan analysis could also enable ultra-low field computed tomography, which makes use of even smaller radiation doses than LDCT.[122] These scans are typically too noisy to discern small pulmonary nodules, but machine learning algorithms can assist with denoising the images.

Machine learning-leveraged image analysis can also create novel types of information. For example, author Dr Sequist and colleagues developed a deep learning model called Sybil that analyzes a single LDCT to predict lung cancer risk over the subsequent 6 years.[123] As with many machine learning algorithms, it is unclear which features Sybil is extracting to generate these predictions, but it is quite accurate, with a 6-year ROC of 0.75 to 0.81, and has been validated in 3 independent populations to date. Another lung cancer prediction model by Ardila and colleagues first detects individual lesions and then uses the regions of interest along with the full LDCT volume to predict 1- and 2-year cancer risk, achieving ROC-AUCs of 0.944 and 0.873, respectively.[117] These and other algorithms could inform personalized screening intervals, with higher risk individuals returning for screening LDCTs more frequently than lower risk individuals.[124] Moreover, such algorithms could have an essential role in identifying those most at risk for lung cancer, including those who are not currently eligible for screening.

Novel screening tools are in development that could become essential complements to LDCT or perhaps even supplant LDCT. In general, these tools detect traces of cancer by-products from easily sampled media like blood, exhaled breath, stool, and even urine.[111–114] Some of these tests are designed to detect dozens of cancers at once, whereas others are optimized for single cancer detection. Clinical trials are ongoing to determine which tests are most informative. Most recently, the PATH-FINDER and SYMPLIFY trials described the performance of Galleri, a multi-cancer detection blood test in asymptomatic and symptomatic individuals, respectively.[114,125] In asymptomatic individuals, 1.4% received a positive test, of which approximately 40% were true positives. Currently, no data have yet suggested that these tests result in a stage shift at diagnosis or an overall survival improvement. But these assays hold the promise of high throughput, convenient tests that could help make cancer screening more accessible, particularly in rural and other under-resourced areas in the US and globally.

SUMMARY

Therapeutics and techniques to treat lung cancer have significantly improved over the past few decades, and high cure rates are now possible if lung cancer iscaught at an early stage. Unfortunately, without LCS, lung cancer tends to present at an advanced stage, and hence it remains the number one cancer killer in the US and worldwide. Screening asymptomatic individuals with LDCT has tremendous potential to greatly increase early stage lung cancer detection and reduce lung cancer mortality. While the benefit of LCS has been proven in several large-scale randomized trials and is now endorsed by both the USPSTF and CMS, US implementation of lung screening continues to fall far short of its potential. Moreover, current eligibility criteria exclude many at-risk individuals. Indeed, less than half of patients diagnosed with lung cancer would have qualified for screening, with eligibility rates even lower among those who are non-white and female. To solve these injustices, we as a field must improve screening eligibility criteria to be more comprehensive and equitable, and we must revise policies to make screening more accessible and affordable. Lung cancer screening should be as widespread and accessible as breast, colon, and cervical screening.

CLINICS CARE POINTS

- Lung cancer screening of high-risk patients is associated with a 20% improvement in lung cancer mortality and a 6% improvement in all-cause mortality.
- Current LCS guidelines in the US recommend patients aged 50 years to 80 years with at least a 20 pack-year history of tobacco use and who are either currently using tobacco or quit within 15 years undergo annual LDCT

DISCLOSURE

Dr L.V. Sequist receives institutional research support from AstraZeneca, United Kindom, Novartis, Switzerland, Delfi Diagnostics, United States, and participates in a clinical demonstration project funded by Grail, United States.

REFERENCES

1. SEER*Explorer: An interactive website for SEER cancer statistics [Internet]. Surveillance Research Program, National Cancer Institute; 2024. Available at: https://seer.cancer.gov/statistics-network/explorer/. Accessed April 28, 2024.
2. American Cancer Society. Cancer facts & figures 2023. Atlanta, GA: American Cancer Society, Inc.; 2023.
3. Chansky K, Detterbeck FC, Nicholson AG, et al. The IASLC Lung Cancer Staging Project: External Validation of the Revision of the TNM Stage Groupings in the Eighth Edition of the TNM Classification of Lung Cancer. J Thorac Oncol 2017;12:1109–21.
4. Forde PM, Spicer J, Lu S, et al. Neoadjuvant nivolumab plus chemotherapy in resectable lung cancer. N Engl J Med 2022;386:1973–85.
5. Felip E, Altorki N, Zhou C, et al. Adjuvant atezolizumab after adjuvant chemotherapy in resected stage IB-IIIA non-small-cell lung cancer (IMpower010): a randomised, multicentre, open-label, phase 3 trial. Lancet 2021;398:1344–57.

6. Wakelee H, Liberman M, Kato T, et al. Perioperative Pembrolizumab for Early-Stage Non-Small-Cell Lung Cancer. N Engl J Med 2023;389:491–503.

7. Tsuboi M, Herbst RS, John T, et al. Overall Survival with Osimertinib in Resected *EGFR*-Mutated NSCLC. N Engl J Med 2023;389(2):137–47.

8. Ahn JS, Wu Y-L, Dziadziuszko R, et al. LBA1 Efficacy and safety of adjuvant alectinib vs platinum-based chemotherapy (CT) in patients (pts) from Asia with resected, early-stage ALK+ non-small cell lung cancer (NSCLC): a sub analysis of ALINA. Madrid, Spain: European Society of Medical Oncology; 2023. p. S1646–7.

9. Altorki N, Wang X, Kozono D, et al. Lobar or sublobar resection for peripheral stage IA non-small-cell lung cancer. N Engl J Med 2023;388:489–98.

10. Poon C, Wilsdon T, Sarwar I, et al. Why is the screening rate in lung cancer still low? A seven-country analysis of the factors affecting adoption. Front Public Health 2023;11:1264342.

11. Buchberger DS, Videtic GMM. Stereotactic body radiotherapy for the management of early-stage non-small-cell lung cancer: a clinical overview. JCO Oncol Pract 2023;19:239–49.

12. American Lung Association: American Lung Association State of Lung Cancer 2023. Chicago, IL, 2023. Available at: https://www.lung.org/research/state-of-lung-cancer/key-findings.

13. Hall IJ, Tangka FKL, Sabatino SA, et al. Patterns and trends in cancer screening in the United States. Prev Chronic Dis 2018;15:E97.

14. Osarogiagbon RU, Yang PC, Sequist LV. Expanding the reach and grasp of lung cancer screening. Am Soc Clin Oncol Educ Book 2023;43:e389958.

15. Weiss W, Boucot KR, Seidman H. The Philadelphia pulmonary neoplasms research project. Clin Chest Med 1982;3:243–56.

16. Dales LG, Friedman GD, Collen MF. Evaluating periodic multiphasic health checkups: a controlled trial. J Chronic Dis 1979;32:385–404.

17. Brett GZ. Earlier diagnosis and survival in lung cancer. Br Med J 1969;4:260–2.

18. Nash FA, Morgan JM, Tomkins JG. South London Lung Cancer Study. Br Med J 1968;2:715–21.

19. An evaluation of radiologic and cytologic screening for the early detection of lung cancer: a cooperative pilot study of the American Cancer Society and the Veterans Administration. Cancer Res 1966;26:2083–121.

20. Muhm JR, Miller WE, Fontana RS, et al. Lung cancer detected during a screening program using four-month chest radiographs. Radiology 1983;148:609–15.

21. Heelan RT, Flehinger BJ, Melamed MR, et al. Non-small-cell lung cancer: results of the New York screening program. Radiology 1984;151:289–93.

22. Doria-Rose VP, Marcus PM, Szabo E, et al. Randomized controlled trials of the efficacy of lung cancer screening by sputum cytology revisited: a combined mortality analysis from the Johns Hopkins Lung Project and the Memorial Sloan-Kettering Lung Study. Cancer 2009;115:5007–17.

23. Oken MM, Hocking WG, Kvale PA, et al. Screening by chest radiograph and lung cancer mortality: the Prostate, Lung, Colorectal, and Ovarian (PLCO) randomized trial. JAMA 2011;306:1865–73.

24. Henschke CI, McCauley DI, Yankelevitz DF, et al. Early Lung Cancer Action Project: overall design and findings from baseline screening. Lancet 1999;354:99–105.

25. Aberle DR, Adams AM, Berg CD, et al. Reduced lung-cancer mortality with low-dose computed tomographic screening. N Engl J Med 2011;365:395–409.

26. Infante M, Cavuto S, Lutman FR, et al. Long-Term Follow-up Results of the DANTE Trial, a randomized study of lung cancer screening with spiral computed tomography. Am J Respir Crit Care Med 2015;191:1166–75.
27. Pedersen JH, Ashraf H, Dirksen A, et al. The Danish randomized lung cancer CT screening trial–overall design and results of the prevalence round. J Thorac Oncol 2009;4:608–14.
28. Pastorino U, Silva M, Sestini S, et al. Prolonged lung cancer screening reduced 10-year mortality in the MILD trial: new confirmation of lung cancer screening efficacy. Ann Oncol 2019;30:1162–9.
29. de Koning HJ, van der Aalst CM, de Jong PA, et al. Reduced lung-cancer mortality with volume CT screening in a randomized trial. N Engl J Med 2020;382:503–13.
30. Sands J, Tammemagi MC, Couraud S, et al. Lung screening benefits and challenges: a review of the data and outline for implementation. J Thorac Oncol 2021;16:37–53.
31. Hoffman RM, Atallah RP, Struble RD, et al. Lung cancer screening with low-dose CT: a meta-analysis. J Gen Intern Med 2020;35:3015–25.
32. Moyer VA, Force USPST. Screening for lung cancer: U.S. Preventive Services Task Force recommendation statement. Ann Intern Med 2014;160:330–8.
33. Center for Medicare & Medicaid Services HaHS: Centers for Medicare and Medicaid Services Decision memo for screening for lung cancer with low dose computed tomography (LDCT) (CAG-00439N). 2015. Available at: https://www.cms.gov/medicare-coverage-database/view/ncacal-decision-memo.aspx?proposed=N&NCAId=274.
34. Roth JA, Sullivan SD, Goulart BH, et al. Projected clinical, resource use, and fiscal impacts of implementing low-dose computed tomography lung cancer screening in medicare. J Oncol Pract 2015;11:267–72.
35. Silvestri GA, Goldman L, Tanner NT, et al. Outcomes from more than 1 million people screened for lung cancer with low-dose CT imaging. Chest 2023. https://doi.org/10.1016/j.chest.2023.02.003.
36. Humphrey L, Deffebach M, Pappas M, et al. Screening for Lung Cancer: Systematic Review to Update the U.S. Preventive Services Task Force Recommendation. U.S. Preventive Services Task Force Evidence Syntheses, formerly Systematic Evidence Reviews. Rockville, MD, 2013. Available at: https://www.ncbi.nlm.nih.gov/books/NBK154610/.
37. Bach PB, Mirkin JN, Oliver TK, et al. Benefits and harms of CT screening for lung cancer: a systematic review. JAMA 2012;307:2418–29.
38. Pinsky PF, Berg CD. Applying the National Lung Screening Trial eligibility criteria to the US population: what percent of the population and of incident lung cancers would be covered? J Med Screen 2012;19:154–6.
39. Gould MK, Donington J, Lynch WR, et al. Evaluation of individuals with pulmonary nodules: when is it lung cancer? Diagnosis and management of lung cancer, 3rd ed: American College of Chest Physicians evidence-based clinical practice guidelines. Chest 2013;143:e93S–120S.
40. Callister ME, Baldwin DR, Akram AR, et al. British Thoracic Society guidelines for the investigation and management of pulmonary nodules. Thorax 2015;70(Suppl 2):ii1–54.
41. Prosper AE, Kammer MN, Maldonado F, et al. Expanding role of advanced image analysis in CT-detected indeterminate pulmonary nodules and early lung cancer characterization. Radiology 2023;309:e222904.

42. MacMahon H, Austin JH, Gamsu G, et al. Guidelines for management of small pulmonary nodules detected on CT scans: a statement from the Fleischner Society. Radiology 2005;237:395–400.

43. Swensen SJ, Silverstein MD, Ilstrup DM, et al. The probability of malignancy in solitary pulmonary nodules. Application to small radiologically indeterminate nodules. Arch Intern Med 1997;157:849–55.

44. McWilliams A, Tammemagi MC, Mayo JR, et al. Probability of cancer in pulmonary nodules detected on first screening CT. N Engl J Med 2013;369:910–9.

45. Roberts TJ, Lennes IT, Hawari S, et al. Integrated, multidisciplinary management of pulmonary nodules can streamline care and improve adherence to recommendations. Oncol 2020;25:431–7.

46. LeMense GP, Waller EA, Campbell C, et al. Development and outcomes of a comprehensive multidisciplinary incidental lung nodule and lung cancer screening program. BMC Pulm Med 2020;20:115.

47. Mankidy BJ, Mohammad G, Trinh K, et al. High risk lung nodule: A multidisciplinary approach to diagnosis and management. Respir Med 2023;214:107277.

48. Milligan MG, Lennes IT, Hawari S, et al. Incidence of radiation therapy among patients enrolled in a multidisciplinary pulmonary nodule and lung cancer screening clinic. JAMA Netw Open 2022;5:e224840.

49. Kumar AJ, Tran DH, Sivasailam B, et al. The effect of a dedicated lung mass clinic on lung nodule follow up. Ann Public Health Epidemiol 2022;1.

50. Madariaga ML, Lennes IT, Best T, et al. Multidisciplinary selection of pulmonary nodules for surgical resection: Diagnostic results and long-term outcomes. J Thorac Cardiovasc Surg 2020;159:1558–1566 e3.

51. Osarogiagbon RU, Liao W, Faris NR, et al. Lung cancer diagnosed through screening, lung nodule, and neither program: a prospective observational study of the Detecting Early Lung Cancer (DELUGE) in the Mississippi Delta Cohort. J Clin Oncol 2022;40:2094–105.

52. Osarogiagbon RU, Liao W, Faris NR, et al. Evaluation of lung cancer risk among persons undergoing screening or guideline-concordant monitoring of lung nodules in the Mississippi Delta. JAMA Netw Open 2023;6:e230787.

53. Association AL: New Study from American Lung Association's Lung Force Reveals Low Awareness of Lifesaving Lung Cancer Screening among Those at Greatest Risk, 2023. https://www.lung.org/media/press-releases/new-study-lung-cancer-screening.

54. Schiffelbein JE, Carluzzo KL, Hasson RM, et al. Barriers, facilitators, and suggested interventions for lung cancer screening among a rural screening-eligible population. J Prim Care Community Health 2020;11. 2150132720930544.

55. Sahar L, Douangchai Wills VL, Liu KKA, et al. Geographic access to lung cancer screening among eligible adults living in rural and urban environments in the United States. Cancer 2022;128:1584–94.

56. Cavers D, Nelson M, Rostron J, et al. Understanding patient barriers and facilitators to uptake of lung screening using low dose computed tomography: a mixed methods scoping review of the current literature. Respir Res 2022;23:374.

57. Martinez MC, Stults CD, Li J. Provider and patient perspectives to improve lung cancer screening with low-dose computed tomography 5 years after Medicare coverage: a qualitative study. BMC Prim Care 2022;23:332.

58. Khanna A, Fix GM, McCullough MB, et al. Implementing shared decision-making for lung cancer screening across a Veterans Health Administration Hospital Network: a hybrid effectiveness-implementation study protocol. Ann Am Thorac Soc 2022;19:476–83.

59. Rivera MP, Katki HA, Tanner NT, et al. Addressing disparities in lung cancer screening eligibility and healthcare access. an official American Thoracic Society Statement. Am J Respir Crit Care Med 2020;202:e95–112.

60. Tanner NT, Silvestri GA. Shared decision-making and lung cancer screening: let's get the conversation started. Chest 2019;155:21–4.

61. Lee SJC, Lee J, Zhu H, et al. Assessing barriers and facilitators to lung cancer screening: initial findings from a patient navigation intervention. Popul Health Manag 2023;26:177–84.

62. Stowell JT, Narayan AK, Wang GX, et al. Factors affecting patient adherence to lung cancer screening: A multisite analysis. J Med Screen 2021;28:357–64.

63. Tanner NT, Brasher PB, Wojciechowski B, et al. Screening adherence in the veterans administration lung cancer screening demonstration project. Chest 2020; 158:1742–52.

64. Lopez-Olivo MA, Maki KG, Choi NJ, et al. Patient adherence to screening for lung cancer in the US: A systematic review and meta-analysis. JAMA Netw Open 2020;3:e2025102.

65. Loomis D, Grosse Y, Lauby-Secretan B, et al. The carcinogenicity of outdoor air pollution. Lancet Oncol 2013;14:1262–3.

66. Hill W, Lim EL, Weeden CE, et al. Lung adenocarcinoma promotion by air pollutants. Nature 2023;616:159–67.

67. Berg CD, Schiller JH, Boffetta P, et al. Air pollution and lung cancer: a review by International Association for the Study of Lung Cancer Early Detection and Screening Committee. J Thorac Oncol 2023;18:1277–89.

68. Li T, Kung HJ, Mack PC, et al. Genotyping and genomic profiling of non-small-cell lung cancer: implications for current and future therapies. J Clin Oncol 2013; 31:1039–49.

69. Vigneswaran J, Tan YH, Murgu SD, et al. Comprehensive genetic testing identifies targetable genomic alterations in most patients with non-small cell lung cancer, specifically adenocarcinoma, single institute investigation. Oncotarget 2016;7:18876–86.

70. Kim ES, Roy UB, Ersek JL, et al. Updates regarding biomarker testing for non-small cell lung cancer: considerations from the National Lung Cancer Roundtable. J Thorac Oncol 2019;14:338–42.

71. Sorscher S, LoPiccolo J, Heald B, et al. Rate of pathogenic germline variants in patients with lung cancer. JCO Precis Oncol 2023;7:e2300190.

72. Scagliotti GV, Longo M, Novello S. Nonsmall cell lung cancer in never smokers. Curr Opin Oncol 2009;21:99–104.

73. Pelosof L, Ahn C, Gao A, et al. Proportion of never-smoker non-small cell lung cancer patients at three diverse institutions. J Natl Cancer Inst 2017;109.

74. Cufari ME, Proli C, De Sousa P, et al. Increasing frequency of non-smoking lung cancer: Presentation of patients with early disease to a tertiary institution in the UK. Eur J Cancer 2017;84:55–9.

75. Carter-Harris L, Gould MK. Multilevel barriers to the successful implementation of lung cancer screening: why does it have to be so hard? Ann Am Thorac Soc 2017;14:1261–5.

76. Delmerico J, Hyland A, Celestino P, et al. Patient willingness and barriers to receiving a CT scan for lung cancer screening. Lung Cancer 2014;84:307–9.

77. Zeliadt SB, Hoffman RM, Birkby G, et al. Challenges implementing lung cancer screening in federally qualified health centers. Am J Prev Med 2018;54:568–75.

78. Kukhareva PV, Caverly TJ, Li H, et al. Inaccuracies in electronic health records smoking data and a potential approach to address resulting underestimation in

determining lung cancer screening eligibility. J Am Med Inform Assoc 2022;29: 779–88.

79. Modin HE, Fathi JT, Gilbert CR, et al. Pack-year cigarette smoking history for determination of lung cancer screening eligibility. comparison of the electronic medical record versus a shared decision-making conversation. Ann Am Thorac Soc 2017;14:1320–5.
80. Haddad DN, Sandler KL, Henderson LM, et al. Disparities in lung cancer screening: a review. Ann Am Thorac Soc 2020;17:399–405.
81. Raman V, Yong V, Erkmen CP, et al. Social disparities in lung cancer risk and screening. Thorac Surg Clin 2022;32:23–31.
82. Potter AL, Senthil P, Srinivasan D, et al. Persistent racial and sex-based disparities in lung cancer screening eligibility. J Thorac Cardiovasc Surg 2023. https://doi.org/10.1016/j.jtcvs.2023.10.025.
83. Rustagi AS, Byers AL, Brown JK, et al. Lung Cancer Screening Among U.S. Military Veterans by Health Status and Race and Ethnicity, 2017-2020: A Cross-Sectional Population-Based Study. AJPM Focus 2023;2:100084.
84. Fiscella K, Winters P, Farah S, et al. Do lung cancer eligibility criteria align with risk among blacks and hispanics? PLoS One 2015;10:e0143789.
85. Pasquinelli MM, Tammemagi MC, Kovitz KL, et al. Risk prediction model versus united states preventive services task force lung cancer screening eligibility criteria: reducing race disparities. J Thorac Oncol 2020;15:1738–47.
86. Force USPST, Krist AH, Davidson KW, et al. Screening for lung cancer: US Preventive Services Task Force Recommendation Statement. JAMA 2021;325: 962–70.
87. Pinheiro LC, Groner L, Soroka O, et al. Analysis of eligibility for lung cancer screening by race after 2021 Changes to US Preventive Services Task Force Screening Guidelines. JAMA Netw Open 2022;5:e2229741.
88. Shusted CS, Evans NR, Kane GC, et al. Analysis of lung cancer screening by race after USPSTF Expansion of Screening Eligibility in 2021. JAMA Netw Open 2022;5:e2217578.
89. Pu CY, Lusk CM, Neslund-Dudas C, et al. Comparison between the 2021 USPSTF lung cancer screening criteria and other lung cancer screening criteria for racial disparity in eligibility. JAMA Oncol 2022;8:374–82.
90. Choi E, Ding VY, Luo SJ, et al. Risk model-based lung cancer screening and racial and ethnic disparities in the US. JAMA Oncol 2023;9:1640–8.
91. Narayan AK, Chowdhry DN, Fintelmann FJ, et al. Racial and ethnic disparities in lung cancer screening eligibility. Radiology 2021;301:712–20.
92. Aredo JV, Choi E, Ding VY, et al. Racial and ethnic disparities in lung cancer screening by the 2021 USPSTF guidelines versus risk-based criteria: the multi-ethnic cohort study. JNCI Cancer Spectr 2022;6.
93. Potter AL, Yang CJ, Woolpert KM, et al. Evaluating eligibility of US Black Women Under USPSTF Lung Cancer Screening Guidelines. JAMA Oncol 2022;8:163–4.
94. Liu A, Siddiqi N, Tapan U, et al. Black race remains associated with lower eligibility for screening using 2021 US Preventive Services Task Force Recommendations Among Lung Cancer Patients at an Urban Safety Net Hospital. J Racial Ethn Health Disparities 2023;10:2836–43.
95. Smeltzer MP, Liao W, Faris NR, et al. Potential impact of criteria modifications on race and sex disparities in eligibility for lung cancer screening. J Thorac Oncol 2023;18:158–68.
96. Pasquinelli MM, Tammemagi MC, Kovitz KL, et al. Brief report: risk prediction model versus united states preventive services task force 2020 draft lung

cancer screening eligibility criteria-reducing race disparities. JTO Clin Res Rep 2021;2:100137.

97. Pinsky PF, Zhu CS, Kramer BS. Lung cancer risk by years since quitting in 30+ pack year smokers. J Med Screen 2015;22:151–7.

98. Kondo KK, Rahman B, Ayers CK, et al. Lung cancer diagnosis and mortality beyond 15 years since quit in individuals with a 20+ pack-year history: A systematic review. CA Cancer J Clin 2023. https://doi.org/10.3322/caac.21808.

99. Wolf AMD, Oeffinger KC, Shih TY, et al. Screening for lung cancer: 2023 guideline update from the American Cancer Society. CA Cancer J Clin 2023. https://doi.org/10.3322/caac.21811.

100. Potter AL, Xu NN, Senthil P, et al. Pack-year smoking history: An inadequate and biased measure to determine lung cancer screening eligibility. J Clin Oncol 2024. JCO 2301780.

101. Kim YH, Warren SH, Kooter I, et al. Chemistry, lung toxicity and mutagenicity of burn pit smoke-related particulate matter. Part Fibre Toxicol 2021;18:45.

102. Grier W, Abbas H, Gebeyehu RR, et al. Military exposures and lung cancer in United States veterans. Semin Oncol 2022. https://doi.org/10.1053/j.seminoncol.2022.06.010.

103. Kerpel-Fronius A, Tammemagi M, Cavic M, et al. Screening for lung cancer in individuals who never smoked: An International Association for the Study of Lung Cancer Early Detection and Screening Committee Report. J Thorac Oncol 2022;17:56–66.

104. Potter AL, Rosenstein AL, Kiang MV, et al. Association of computed tomography screening with lung cancer stage shift and survival in the United States: quasi-experimental study. BMJ 2022;376:e069008.

105. Khouzam MS, Wood DE, Vigneswaran W, et al. Impact of Federal Lung Cancer Screening Policy on the Incidence of Early-stage Lung Cancer. Ann Thorac Surg 2023;115:827–33.

106. Ganti AK, Klein AB, Cotarla I, et al. Update of incidence, prevalence, survival, and initial treatment in patients with non-small cell lung cancer in the US. JAMA Oncol 2021;7:1824–32.

107. Flores R, Patel P, Alpert N, et al. Association of stage shift and population mortality among patients with non-small cell lung cancer. JAMA Netw Open 2021;4:e2137508.

108. Pua BB, O'Neill BC, Ortiz AK, et al. Results from lung cancer screening outreach utilizing a mobile CT Scanner in an Urban Area. J Am Coll Radiol 2023. https://doi.org/10.1016/j.jacr.2023.10.025.

109. Raghavan D, Wheeler M, Doege D, et al. Initial results from mobile low-dose computerized tomographic lung cancer screening unit: improved outcomes for underserved populations. Oncol 2020;25:e777–81.

110. Adams SJ, Stone E, Baldwin DR, et al. Lung cancer screening. Lancet 2023;401:390–408.

111. Ulz P, Perakis S, Zhou Q, et al. Inference of transcription factor binding from cell-free DNA enables tumor subtype prediction and early detection. Nat Commun 2019;10:4666.

112. Mathios D, Johansen JS, Cristiano S, et al. Detection and characterization of lung cancer using cell-free DNA fragmentomes. Nat Commun 2021;12:5060.

113. Meng S, Li Q, Zhou Z, et al. Assessment of an exhaled breath test using high-pressure photon ionization time-of-flight mass spectrometry to detect lung cancer. JAMA Netw Open 2021;4:e213486.

114. Schrag D, Beer TM, McDonnell CH 3rd, et al. Blood-based tests for multicancer early detection (PATHFINDER): a prospective cohort study. Lancet 2023;402: 1251–60.
115. Adams SJ, Mondal P, Penz E, et al. Development and cost analysis of a lung nodule management strategy combining artificial intelligence and lung-RADS for baseline lung cancer screening. J Am Coll Radiol 2021;18:741–51.
116. Setio AAA, Traverso A, de Bel T, et al. Validation, comparison, and combination of algorithms for automatic detection of pulmonary nodules in computed tomography images: The LUNA16 challenge. Med Image Anal 2017;42:1–13.
117. Ardila D, Kiraly AP, Bharadwaj S, et al. End-to-end lung cancer screening with three-dimensional deep learning on low-dose chest computed tomography. Nat Med 2019;25:954–61.
118. Cui X, Zheng S, Heuvelmans MA, et al. Performance of a deep learning-based lung nodule detection system as an alternative reader in a Chinese lung cancer screening program. Eur J Radiol 2022;146:110068.
119. Hawkins S, Wang H, Liu Y, et al. Predicting malignant nodules from screening CT scans. J Thorac Oncol 2016;11:2120–8.
120. Huang P, Lin CT, Li Y, et al. Prediction of lung cancer risk at follow-up screening with low-dose CT: a training and validation study of a deep learning method. Lancet Digit Health 2019;1:e353–62.
121. Adams SJ, Madtes DK, Burbridge B, et al. Clinical impact and generalizability of a computer-assisted diagnostic tool to risk-stratify lung nodules with CT. J Am Coll Radiol 2023;20:232–42.
122. Hata A, Yanagawa M, Yoshida Y, et al. Combination of deep learning-based denoising and iterative reconstruction for ultra-low-dose CT of the chest: image quality and lung-RADS evaluation. AJR Am J Roentgenol 2020;215:1321–8.
123. Mikhael PG, Wohlwend J, Yala A, et al. Sybil: a validated deep learning model to predict future lung cancer risk from a single low-dose chest computed tomography. J Clin Oncol 2023. https://doi.org/10.1200/JCO.22.01345. JCO2201345.
124. Silvestri GA, Jett JR. The intersection of lung cancer screening, radiomics, and artificial intelligence: can one scan really predict the future development of lung cancer? J Clin Oncol 2023;41:2141–3.
125. Nicholson BD, Oke J, Virdee PS, et al. Multi-cancer early detection test in symptomatic patients referred for cancer investigation in England and Wales (SYMPLIFY): a large-scale, observational cohort study. Lancet Oncol 2023;24: 733–43.

Cervical Cancer
Precursors and Prevention

Vikrant V. Sahasrabuddhe, MBBS, MPH, DrPH

KEYWORDS

- Cervical cancer • Human papillomavirus (HPV) • Screening • Vaccines • Testing
- Pap smears • Self-collection • Screen-and-treat

KEY POINTS

- Cervical cancer precursors, sequelae of persistent, oncogenic human papillomavirus (HPV) infection, can progress to invasive cervical cancer if left undetected and untreated.
- Primary or adjunctive screening with molecular HPV testing offers high clinical sensitivity for detection of cervical cancer precursors over cervical cytology ('Papanicolaou test').
- Scaling up of HPV prophylactic vaccination and increasing prevention access to under-screened populations globally can substantially reduce the public health burden of cervical cancer.

INTRODUCTION AND EPIDEMIOLOGY

Cervical cancer is a leading cause of cancer-related morbidity and mortality worldwide. Over 660,000 women are diagnosed, and over 348,000 die every year, due to cervical cancer.[1] Cervical cancer remains one of the most common and most deadly malignances among women, particularly in low-income and middle-income countries globally, where it is often one of the leading or second-leading causes of cancer-related cases and deaths.[2] Cervical cancer primarily affects women between the third and fifth decades of their lives and has significant intergenerational impact due to millions of children orphaned and families and societies destabilized in its wake.[3]

Chronic persistent infection with oncogenic human papillomavirus (HPV) has been identified as the obligate cause of cervical cancer.[4] HPV is a very common sexually transmitted infection acquired with the onset of sexual activity, and the vast majority of individuals clear HPV infection on their own.[5] Yet, it persists in the cervical basal epithelial layers for several years in a small fraction of individuals, where it leads to progressive oncogenic cellular changes and asymptomatic sequelae as cervical cancer

Breast and Gynecologic Cancer Research Group, Division of Cancer Prevention, National Cancer Institute, National Institutes of Health, 9609 Medical Center Drive, Room 5E-338, Rockville, MD, USA
E-mail address: vikrant.sahasrabuddhe@nih.gov
Twitter: @iVikVS (V.V.S.)

Hematol Oncol Clin N Am 38 (2024) 771–781
https://doi.org/10.1016/j.hoc.2024.03.005
0889-8588/24/© 2024 Elsevier Inc. All rights reserved, including those for text and data mining, AI training, and similar technologies.

precursors (**Fig. 1**). These lesions, if left undetected and untreated, can lead to eventual invasive changes and symptomatic presentation several years later in an overall small proportion of individuals.[6] There are more than 100 types of HPVs, of which 13 types (called 'high-risk HPV' or 'hrHPV' types) are known to cause cervical cancer, with variable attributable risk.[4] Yet, HPV infection by itself is not a sufficient cause of cervical cancer, and several other factors modulate the carcinogenesis risk.[7] These include age,[8] alterations in the immune status (notably immunosuppression via infectious etiologies like human immunodeficiency virus (HIV)[9] and iatrogenic immunosuppression in transplant recipients[10]), hormonal influences (including higher number of pregnancies, long-term contraceptive use), behavioral factors (including greater

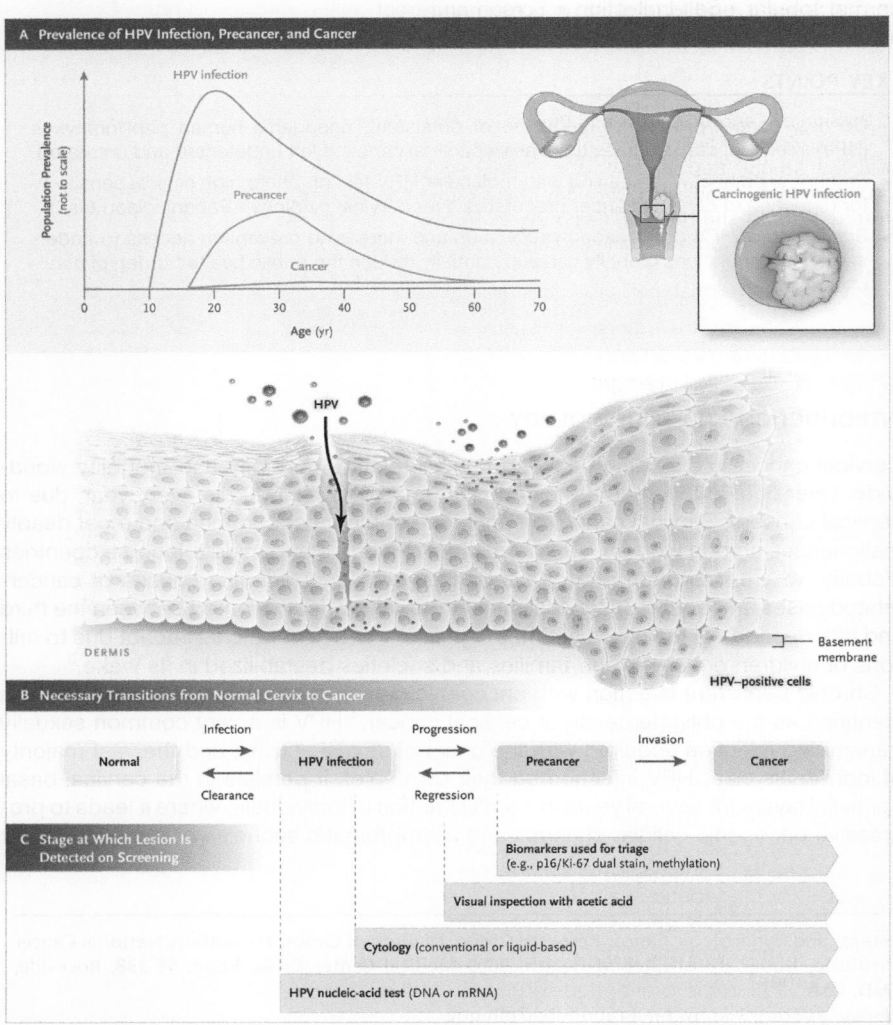

Fig. 1. Schematic representation of the natural history of cervical cancer. DNA, deoxyribonucleic acid; HPV, human papillomavirus; mRNA, messenger ribonucleic acid. (*From*: Bouvard V, Wentzensen N, Mackie A, et al. The IARC Perspective on Cervical Cancer Screening. *N Engl J Med*. Nov 11 2021;385(20):1908–1918, doi:10.1056/NEJMsr2030640; with permission)

number of sexual partners, earlier age at sexual intercourse), smoking, and concurrent sexually transmitted infections, among other factors.[7,11]

The current landscapes of the clinical management of cervical cancer and public health paradigms for its prevention and control are a result of decades-long, multidisciplinary scientific investigations into the etiology, natural history, and pathogenesis of this disease.[12] These efforts have ranged from the characterization of microscopically visible abnormal changes in cervical cells in smears from vaginally collected cervical samples observable for several years before the onset of symptoms[13] to advances in molecular characterization methodologies leading to the discovery of HPV as the viral etiologic agent,[14] as well as key innovations in detection (molecular HPV testing[15]) and prevention (prophylactic HPV vaccination[16]). Consequently, cervical cancer is one of the most preventable of all malignancies, and incidence rates have dropped precipitously in the United States and most higher income countries over the second half of the twentieth century. This reduction is mostly as a result of widespread screening and early detection, and there is emerging evidence about the beneficial impact of prophylactic vaccination on reduction in cervical cancer precursors and cancer incidence, especially as vaccinated cohorts advance in age in the coming decades.[17]

Yet, most women present are diagnosed with cervical cancer at advanced stages when options for prevention and treatment are limited.[18] In particular, access to screening and prevention services remains limited for millions of women globally, including in most low-income and middle-income countries as well as areas of health care inequities in the United States.[19] Individuals with inadequate access to preventive and therapeutic care including those from lower socio-economic backgrounds, races/ ethnicities facing social and structural inequities and historical discrimination, and residents of areas with geographic and physical inaccessibility to health care facilities face higher incidence and mortality rates due to cervical cancer.[20] There are increasing efforts and awareness globally to address such disparities by coordinated global action and targeting the elimination of cervical cancer as a public health problem globally.[1,21]

CERVICAL CANCER PRECURSORS

The vast majority of cervical cancers are squamous cell carcinomas (SCCs) that arise from oncogenic transformation of squamous cells at the cervical transformation zone (junction of the squamous and columnar cell layers of the mucosal epithelium at the cervical opening of the uterus), while the rest are adenocarcinomas and other rarer histologic types. Secondary prevention of cervical cancer screening involves early detection of precancerous lesions (precursors) associated with chronic, persistent HPV infection and treatment of these lesions. Cervical cancer screening primarily involves collection and examination of cervical cells for detection of dysplastic cells ('Papanicolaou test [Pap test]'), as well as testing for oncogenic HPV types ('HPV testing') in the same samples. Individuals with abnormal screening test results are referred for diagnostic evaluation using colposcopy which involves magnified visualization of the cervix and, if necessary, collection of tissue specimens (via cervical biopsy or endocervical curettage) for histopathologic evaluation, followed by management that follows standardized, risk-stratified, consensus-based national and international guidelines.[22,23] The cytologic and histologic precursor lesions for cervical cancer have been characterized with several variations in terminologies that have evolved over time.[24] Reporting of cervical screening results is based on grades of abnormal cytology (eg, mild, moderate, and severe dysplasia; and low-grade and high-grade squamous intraepithelial lesions: LSIL and HSIL, respectively) as well as a plethora of descriptors (eg, atypical squamous cells of undetermined significance) that also rely on integrating results of triage testing or co-testing with molecular HPV testing/HPV genotyping approaches and related descriptors (eg, hrHPV positive, HPV16 positive, HPV18 positive). Histologic reporting has long relied on the use of the 'cervical intraepithelial neoplasia (CIN)' grading terminology, with CIN1, CIN2, and CIN3 as descriptors reflective of the extent of involvement of the full thickness of the squamous epithelium. CIN3 (formerly also referred to as carcinoma in situ) is the most stringently defined precursor of cervical SCCs. Adenocarcinoma in situ is the columnar cell–equivalent precursor for cervical adenocarcinoma. Innovations in immunohistochemical biomarkers (eg, P16, Ki67) of oncogenic cellular transformation due to chronic, persistent HPV infection improve CIN3 risk prediction, and newer histologic reporting guidelines recommend using these biomarkers for secondary testing on intermediate-grade diagnoses (eg, CIN2) for an improved risk-stratified and clinically actionable reporting of histologic reporting categories of LSIL and HSIL.

HUMAN PAPILLOMAVIRUS PROPHYLACTIC VACCINES

Currently available viruslike particle–based recombinant subunit HPV vaccines have been shown to be highly effective and safe for preventing incident and persistent HPV infection and its progression to cervical cancer precursors and cancer. This evidence is borne out both from clinical trial data as well as real-world evidence from registry-linkage and surveillance studies over the past 2 decades.[25] Current vaccines vary in their HPV type coverage (eg, bivalent covers HPV16/18, quadrivalent covers HPV16/18/6/11, and nonavalent covers HPV 16/18/6/11/31/33/45/52/58; the latter covers types responsible for causing over 90% of cervical cancers).[26] These vaccines are prophylactic in nature (ie, prevent acquisition of new type-specific infection, with some cross-type protective efficacy) and most efficacious when given prior to sexual exposure to HPV. Although approved for a broad age range (eg, ages 9–45 years in the United States), most public health recommendations globally emphasize vaccination between 9 and 14 years of age, prior to initiation of sexual activity. Although originally approved as a 3-dose series, emerging global evidence has influenced progressive changes in recommendations for fewer doses, and a recently announced permissive recommendation for single dose schedules for those between 9 and 14 years can rapidly accelerate global targets for vaccine coverage.[27,28] Girls are the primary focus for HPV vaccination with a goal on cervical cancer prevention, but recommendations have also been extended to boys—especially in many high-resource countries, since HPV is also a recognized causative factor for anogenital cancers as well as oropharyngeal cancers.[29]

Although there is clinical interest in the use of HPV prophylactic vaccines after/around the time of treatment of precancerous lesions to prevent recurrences, the mechanism of action of prophylactic vaccines does not suggest a therapeutic effect. And although new infections or autoinoculation with new types may be preventable, there is no definitive clinical trial evidence suggesting lower risk of recurrence of lesions after treatment of cervical cancer precursors. Clinical trials exploring the role of nonavalent HPV vaccination in the peri-treatment setting, including in immunosuppressed individuals with HIV, are currently underway.[30]

SCREENING, MANAGEMENT, AND DIAGNOSIS OF CERVICAL CANCER PRECURSORS

Periodic testing with cervical cytology ('Pap testing') in adult, sexually active women has been the mainstay of cervical cancer screening in higher resource settings globally. Cytology relies on morphologic evaluation of cells, and methods to process and prepare specimens have evolved from conventional slide-based smears ('Pap smears') to liquid-media based cytologic cellular detection, including via automation-aided cell characterization approaches. Over the past 2 decades, several highly sensitive molecular HPV testing approaches that rely on an objective detection of markers such as HPV DNA or messenger RNA, via polymerase chain reaction and related technologies, have been approved for use.[31] These tests are used for triage of abnormal or indeterminate cytology, as a co-test with cytology, or as a primary screening approach (ie, as an alternative to cytology). Screening guidelines have evolved with accumulating evidence about the clinical effectiveness and cost-effectiveness of HPV testing, and now increasingly recommend primary HPV screening as the preferred approach.[32]

Management of positive HPV testing necessitates further risk stratification with genotyping (eg, HPV16 or HPV18 requiring an immediate colposcopy/diagnostic approach vs active surveillance for other hrHPV types) or reflex cytology for immunocytochemical markers (eg, P16/Ki67 dual stain) to provide biologically salient approaches that balance the need for maximized disease detection without overwhelming referrals for colposcopy.[32] Several newer advances such as host and viral methylation markers, oncoprotein testing, and technologies using artificial intelligence/machine learning approaches to improve and automate reflex cytology are being investigated for their accuracy and utility as triage markers in management pathways.[20,33]

HPV testing can also be done on vaginal self-collected samples or on urine samples, thereby providing opportunities for screening without the need for a pelvic examination to collect specimens.[34] This can be a significant advantage for individuals and communities that are unable or unwilling to undergo traditional clinic-based/pelvic examination–based screening due to personal/medical preferences or limitations in health care access.[35] More than half of all new cases of cervical cancer in the United States occur in those who are never screened or are inadequately screened. Since any potential decrement in detection due to self-collection (due to inherent technical and operational limitations in sampling/transport/processing) could be offset by increased rates of screening uptake (due to the convenience and ease of self-collection approaches), regulatory bodies and public health agencies globally are increasingly looking at innovations and improvements in self-collection approaches as alternatives to expand population-level screening coverage.[34,36]

Many lower resource settings globally lack adequate human resources for implementing complex, multi-visit cytology-based screening programs. This has stimulated investigations into the development of setting-appropriate, lower cost, and point-of-care approaches like 'visual inspection with acetic acid' that provides immediate results and can link screening to diagnostic and treatment interventions in the same visit.[37] Yet, they have significant limitations in accuracy (ie, both higher false-negative and false-positive results) and reproducibility and require significant training and quality assurance efforts.[38] Several promising technologies for point-of-care HPV detection, novel biomarkers for triage of abnormal HPV positive results, and technologies using artificial intelligence/machine learning approaches to augment visual evaluation are on the horizon and if proven effective, may lead to substantial improvements in improving implementation options in lower resource settings globally.[39,40]

Cervical cancer precursors detected via a screening test require diagnostic confirmation, most often done via a magnified visualization with colposcopy.[41] Although several standardized terminologies exist, the inherent subjectivity in human impressions leads to high interobserver variation in colposcopic results.[42] Colposcopy guidelines routinely recommend taking multiple biopsy/tissues samples of visible lesions to maximize the detection of the underlying disease.[43] Novel imaging approaches relying on artificial intelligence/machine learning are being utilized for improvements in colposcopic diagnoses and aiding in the delineation of abnormal areas that need histologic confirmation.[44] Given involution of the cervical transformation zone into the endocervical canal with age-related and menopause-related changes, innovative and alternative colposcopic visualization and tissue sampling approaches have been utilized to further maximize disease detection.[45,46] However, like most human interpretations, histopathologic diagnoses are also subject to wide interobserver variation.[47] Novel immunohistochemical biomarkers (eg, P16, Ki67) that improve risk stratification potential of histologic diagnoses, compared to regular hematoxylin/eosin staining alone, have been used, particularly for intermediate-grade histology (eg, CIN2).[48,49] Several innovations including the use of artificial intelligence/machine learning–based approaches have also been utilized for augmenting the accuracy of immunohistochemistry-based diagnoses.[50]

TREATMENT OF CERVICAL CANCER PRECURSORS

Interventions targeting the removal of cervical cancer precursors that are diagnosed via cervical cancer screening are the mainstay for preventing their progression to cervical cancer. The availability of precancer treatment interventions is both training-dependent and resource-dependent, and several innovations and evolutions in guidelines have been implemented over the past decades.[49,51] Most high-resource setting guidelines emphasize the use of highly efficacious interventions for wide excision of higher grade lesions via large loop excision of the transformation zone/loop electrosurgical excision procedure that can be done in an outpatient clinical setting under local anesthesia.[52] Excision may also be done via cervical conization (also referred to as cold knife conization or cone biopsy) or surgical removal of the cervix (trachelectomy) or the entire uterus (hysterectomy), all of which are inpatient procedures that require general anesthesia. Excisional procedures provide the benefit of yielding tissue samples for histopathology evaluation from the excised specimen, thereby providing additional diagnostic confirmation (than just the histologic diagnosis during the initial colposcopic biopsy/endocervical curettage). Excisional biopsy results are also helpful to predict recurrence or cure based on the evaluation of the completeness of the margin status of the precursor lesions removed during the excisional procedure. In contrast to excisional procedures, ablative approaches such as cryoablation (cryotherapy), thermal ablation ('cold coagulation'), and laser ablation induce local tissue necrosis and are relatively easier, quicker, safe, and less burdensome (ie, without local anesthesia), especially for lower grade and smaller lesions.[53] However, these procedures are also associated with higher rates of recurrence, likely due to lower depth of necrosis and variations in application time and the extent of coverage of lesions.[53] Another disadvantage is the lack of tissue specimens for confirmatory histopathology. Despite their limitations, ablative approaches provide useful intervention opportunities in cervical cancer prevention programs in lower resource settings that rely on a 'screen-and-treat' paradigm that emphasizes a single-visit approach.[15] Such an approach combines a visual inspection–based or a point-of-care HPV testing–based screening result and an ablation procedure for a visual/molecular screen-positive individual without an intermediate diagnostic confirmation step.[54] Efforts in lower resource settings have shown that such an approach can reduce cervical cancer incidence, especially when compared to no screening as an alternative.[49]

Despite their efficacy, cervical precursor treatment approaches are also associated with several common side effects including vaginal bleeding, infection, and foul smelling discharge, among others, most of which can be managed with appropriate care.[55]

Rarer side effects include vaginal and lower urinary tract injury and longer term sequelae such as cervical stenosis, infertility, and cervical incompetence (leading to higher relative risks for miscarriages, pre-term delivery, and low birth weight of the infant).[56] These are of particular significance for younger women seeking to realize their reproductive potential after a cervical precursor treatment procedure. Excisional approaches are also harder to implement in lower resource settings globally due to the costs, effort requirements, and health system–level complexities in scaling up such interventions.[57]

There is an unmet need for a medical (ie, non-excisional/non-ablative) approach for cervical precursor treatment, and this is an area of active scientific investigation. Several locally applied, self-administered/clinician-administered, and topically delivered approaches (eg, 5-flurouracil, imiquimod, cidofovir, artesunate) have been investigated in prevention-focused clinical trials with variable efficacy.[58] Several therapeutic HPV vaccines/immunotherapeutic candidate approaches (including those using peptides, proteins, DNA, RNA, viral-vectored vaccines), predominantly based on the HPV E6/E7 antigens, are also under investigation and in early clinical development.[59] Unlike existing prophylactic HPV vaccines, which prevent acquisition of new infections, therapeutic vaccines are primarily targeted to induce regression of HPV-associated precancers and clear existing HPV infection. As these innovative approaches move further into clinical development, evidence on their safety, effectiveness, and durability, as well as their eventual costs and complexity of dosing and delivery, will be key attributes for considering them as components in the prevention intervention continuum for cervical cancer and other HPV-related cancers.[59]

DISCUSSION

Significant advances in knowledge about its etiology and the multitude of intervention options make cervical cancer a highly preventable malignancy.[60] There have been significant efforts to marshal resources and coordinate efforts globally for expanding options for prevention and control, with a target for reducing the burden of cervical cancer and eliminating it as a public health problem in the decades to come. Such efforts include priority setting such as country-level targets of 90% coverage for HPV vaccination for girls, at least 70% coverage for screening of at-risk women, and 90% coverage for appropriate treatment interventions.[61] Only a few countries in the 'global north' are even close to these targets in the coming years, while most countries in the 'global south' face continued challenges due to shrinking resources for public health, human resource constraints, and operational complexities for reaching these targets. This underscores the importance of continued investigations into innovative approaches for prevention and control, as well as innovations in clinical care delivery and program implementation and scale-up.

CLINICS CARE POINTS

- Persistent, oncogenic types of HPV that lead to cellular proliferative changes and asymptomatic sequelae at the uterine cervix (cervical cancer precursors)—that if left undetected and untreated—can progress to invasive cervical cancer over several years.

- Current approaches to screening have transitioned to the use of molecular HPV testing approaches utilized as an adjunct (for triage or co-testing) or an alternative to cytology ('Pap testing').

- Self-collection approaches for HPV testing offer the potential for expansion of screening access and reduce disparities in cervical cancer incidence.
- Prophylactic HPV vaccination is a safe and highly effective tool, has no therapeutic benefit, and has promise to significantly reduce the incidence of cervical cancer worldwide.
- Treatment of screen-detected cervical precursors with excision and ablation are highly effective approaches yet associated with a low but non-trivial risk of adverse short-term and long-term side effects. Nonsurgical approaches for precancer treatment (including therapeutic HPV vaccines and topical/local applications) are under clinical investigation.

DISCLOSURE

The Author has no financial conflicts of interest to disclose. The opinions expressed by the Author are his own and this material should not be interpreted as representing the official viewpoint of the U.S. Department of Health and Human Services, the National Institutes of Health, or the National Cancer Institute.

REFERENCES

1. Singh D, Vignat J, Lorenzoni V, et al. Global estimates of incidence and mortality of cervical cancer in 2020: a baseline analysis of the WHO Global Cervical Cancer Elimination Initiative. Lancet Glob Health 2023;11(2):e197–206.
2. Frick C, Rumgay H, Vignat J, et al. Quantitative estimates of preventable and treatable deaths from 36 cancers worldwide: a population-based study. Lancet Glob Health 2023;11(11):e1700–12.
3. Guida F, Kidman R, Ferlay J, et al. Global and regional estimates of orphans attributed to maternal cancer mortality in 2020. Nat Med 2022;28(12):2563–72.
4. Bouvard V, Baan R, Straif K, et al. A review of human carcinogens–Part B: biological agents. Lancet Oncol 2009;10(4):321–2.
5. Wijstma ES, Jongen VW, Alberts CJ, et al. Approaches to estimating clearance rates for human papillomavirus groupings: a systematic review and real data examples. Epidemiology 2023;34(1):119–30.
6. Schiffman M, Castle PE, Jeronimo J, et al. Human papillomavirus and cervical cancer. Lancet 2007;370(9590):890–907.
7. Schiffman M, Doorbar J, Wentzensen N, et al. Carcinogenic human papillomavirus infection. Nat Rev Dis Primers 2016;2:16086.
8. Gravitt PE, Winer RL. Natural history of HPV infection across the lifespan: role of viral latency. Viruses 2017;9(10). https://doi.org/10.3390/v9100267.
9. Castle PE, Einstein MH, Sahasrabuddhe VV. Cervical cancer prevention and control in women living with human immunodeficiency virus. CA Cancer J Clin 2021; 71(6):505–26.
10. Nailescu C, Ermel AC, Shew ML. Human papillomavirus-related cancer risk for solid organ transplant recipients during adult life and early prevention strategies during childhood and adolescence. Pediatr Transplant 2022;26(7):e14341.
11. de Sanjose S, Brotons M, Pavon MA. The natural history of human papillomavirus infection. Best Pract Res Clin Obstet Gynaecol 2018;47:2–13.
12. Bosch FX, Broker TR, Forman D, et al. Comprehensive control of human papillomavirus infections and related diseases. Vaccine 2013;31(Suppl 7):H1–31.
13. Swanson AA, Pantanowitz L. The evolution of cervical cancer screening. J Am Soc Cytopathol Jan-Feb 2024;13(1):10–5.

14. zur Hausen H. Papillomavirus infections–a major cause of human cancers. Biochim Biophys Acta 1996;1288(2):F55–78.
15. Bouvard V, Wentzensen N, Mackie A, et al. The IARC perspective on cervical cancer screening. N Engl J Med 2021;385(20):1908–18.
16. Schiller JT, Lowy DR. An introduction to virus infections and human cancer. Recent Results Cancer Res 2021;217:1–11.
17. Markowitz LE, Schiller JT. Human papillomavirus vaccines. J Infect Dis 2021; 224(12 Suppl 2):S367–78.
18. Rahangdale L, Teodoro N, Chinula L, et al. Eliminating cervical cancer as a global public health problem requires equitable action. BMJ 2023;383:2978.
19. Siegel RL, Giaquinto AN, Jemal A. Cancer statistics, 2024. CA Cancer J Clin Jan-Feb 2024;74(1):12–49.
20. Einstein MH, Zhou N, Gabor L, et al. Primary human papillomavirus testing and other new technologies for cervical cancer screening. Obstet Gynecol 2023; 142(5):1036–43.
21. Gultekin M, Ramirez PT, Broutet N, et al. World health organization call for action to eliminate cervical cancer globally. Int J Gynecol Cancer 2020;30(4):426–7.
22. Perkins RB, Guido RS, Castle PE, et al. 2019 ASCCP risk-based management consensus guidelines: updates through 2023. J Low Genit Tract Dis 2024; 28(1):3–6.
23. World Health Organization, Special Programme of Research Development and Research Training in Human Reproduction (World Health Organization). WHO guideline for screening and treatment of cervical pre-cancer lesions for cervical cancer prevention. 2nd edition. World Health Organization; 2021. 1 online resource (1 PDF file (xvi, 97 pages)). Available at: https://www.ncbi.nlm.nih.gov/books/NBK572317/.
24. Nayar R, Wilbur DC. The bethesda system for reporting cervical cytology: a historical perspective. Acta Cytol 2017;61(4–5):359–72.
25. Schiller J, Lowy D. Explanations for the high potency of HPV prophylactic vaccines. Vaccine 2018;36(32 Pt A):4768–73.
26. Villa LL, Richtmann R. HPV vaccination programs in LMIC: is it time to optimize schedules and recommendations? J Pediatr (Rio J) 2023;99(Suppl 1):S57–61.
27. Markowitz LE, Drolet M, Lewis RM, et al. Human papillomavirus vaccine effectiveness by number of doses: Updated systematic review of data from national immunization programs. Vaccine 2022;40(37):5413–32.
28. Kreimer AR, Cernuschi T, Rees H, et al. Public health opportunities resulting from sufficient HPV vaccine supply and a single-dose vaccination schedule. J Natl Cancer Inst 2023;115(3):246–9.
29. Rahangdale L, Mungo C, O'Connor S, et al. Human papillomavirus vaccination and cervical cancer risk. BMJ 2022;379:e070115.
30. Reuschenbach M, Doorbar J, Del Pino M, et al. Prophylactic HPV vaccines in patients with HPV-associated diseases and cancer. Vaccine 2023;41(42):6194–205.
31. Arbyn M, Simon M, Peeters E, et al. 2020 list of human papillomavirus assays suitable for primary cervical cancer screening. Clin Microbiol Infect 2021;27(8): 1083–95.
32. Perkins RB, Wentzensen N, Guido RS, et al. Cervical cancer screening: a review. JAMA 2023;330(6):547–58.
33. Litwin TR, Irvin SR, Chornock RL, et al. Infiltrating T-cell markers in cervical carcinogenesis: a systematic review and meta-analysis. Br J Cancer 2021;124(4): 831–41.

34. Arbyn M, Castle PE, Schiffman M, et al. Meta-analysis of agreement/concordance statistics in studies comparing self- vs clinician-collected samples for HPV testing in cervical cancer screening. Int J Cancer 2022;151(2):308–12.

35. Arbyn M, Costa S, Latsuzbaia A, et al. HPV-based cervical cancer screening on self-samples in the netherlands: challenges to reach women and test performance questions. Cancer Epidemiol Biomarkers Prev 2023;32(2):159–63.

36. Sahasrabuddhe VV, Castle PE, Schiffman M, et al. Reply to: comments on "meta-analysis of agreement/concordance statistics in studies comparing self- vs clinician-collected samples for HPV testing in cervical cancer screening". Int J Cancer 2022;151(3):484–7.

37. Mulongo M, Chibwesha CJ. Prevention of cervical cancer in low-resource african settings. Obstet Gynecol Clin North Am 2022;49(4):771–81.

38. Simms KT, Keane A, Nguyen DTN, et al. Benefits, harms and cost-effectiveness of cervical screening, triage and treatment strategies for women in the general population. Nat Med 2023;29(12):3050–8.

39. Taghavi K, Zhao F, Downham L, et al. Molecular triaging options for women testing HPV positive with self-collected samples. Front Oncol 2023;13:1243888.

40. Kundrod KA, Jeronimo J, Vetter B, et al. Toward 70% cervical cancer screening coverage: Technical challenges and opportunities to increase access to human papillomavirus (HPV) testing. PLOS Glob Public Health 2023;3(8):e0001982.

41. Guido R, Perkins RB. Management of abnormal cervical cancer screening test: a risk-based approach. Clin Obstet Gynecol 2023;66(3):478–99.

42. Hariprasad R, Mittal S, Basu P. Role of colposcopy in the management of women with abnormal cytology. CytoJournal 2022;19:40.

43. Wentzensen N, Walker JL, Gold MA, et al. Multiple biopsies and detection of cervical cancer precursors at colposcopy. J Clin Oncol 2015;33(1):83–9.

44. Rossman AH, Reid HW, Pieters MM, et al. Digital health strategies for cervical cancer control in low- and middle-income countries: systematic review of current implementations and gaps in research. J Med Internet Res 2021;23(5):e23350.

45. Winter M, Cestero RM, Burg A, et al. Fabric-based exocervical and endocervical biopsy in comparison with punch biopsy and sharp curettage. J Low Genit Tract Dis 2012;16(2):80–7.

46. Reich O, Pickel H. 100 years of iodine testing of the cervix: A critical review and implications for the future. Eur J Obstet Gynecol Reprod Biol 2021;261:34–40.

47. Reuschenbach M, Wentzensen N, Dijkstra MG, et al. p16INK4a immunohistochemistry in cervical biopsy specimens: A systematic review and meta-analysis of the interobserver agreement. Am J Clin Pathol 2014;142(6):767–72.

48. Castle PE, Adcock R, Cuzick J, et al. Relationships of p16 immunohistochemistry and other biomarkers with diagnoses of cervical abnormalities: implications for last terminology. Arch Pathol Lab Med 2020;144(6):725–34.

49. Darragh TM, Colgan TJ, Cox JT, et al. The lower anogenital squamous terminology standardization project for hpv-associated lesions: background and consensus recommendations from the college of american pathologists and the american society for colposcopy and cervical pathology. J Low Genit Tract Dis 2012;16(3):205–42.

50. Parham GP, Egemen D, Befano B, et al. Validation in Zambia of a cervical screening strategy including HPV genotyping and artificial intelligence (AI)-based automated visual evaluation. Infect Agents Cancer 2023;18(1):61.

51. Shastri SS, Temin S, Almonte M, et al. Secondary prevention of cervical cancer: ASCO resource-stratified guideline update. JCO Glob Oncol 2022;8:e2200217.

52. Kalliala I, Athanasiou A, Veroniki AA, et al. Incidence and mortality from cervical cancer and other malignancies after treatment of cervical intraepithelial neoplasia: a systematic review and meta-analysis of the literature. Ann Oncol 2020;31(2):213–27.
53. Pinder LF, Parham GP, Basu P, et al. Thermal ablation versus cryotherapy or loop excision to treat women positive for cervical precancer on visual inspection with acetic acid test: pilot phase of a randomised controlled trial. Lancet Oncol 2020; 21(1):175–84.
54. Basu P, Taghavi K, Hu SY, et al. Management of cervical premalignant lesions. Curr Probl Cancer Mar-Apr 2018;42(2):129–36.
55. Kyrgiou M, Athanasiou A, Kalliala IEJ, et al. Obstetric outcomes after conservative treatment for cervical intraepithelial lesions and early invasive disease. Cochrane Database Syst Rev 2017;11(11):CD012847.
56. Kyrgiou M, Bowden SJ, Athanasiou A, et al. Morbidity after local excision of the transformation zone for cervical intra-epithelial neoplasia and early cervical cancer. Best Pract Res Clin Obstet Gynaecol 2021;75:10–22.
57. Parham GP, Mwanahamuntu MH, Kapambwe S, et al. Population-level scale-up of cervical cancer prevention services in a low-resource setting: development, implementation, and evaluation of the cervical cancer prevention program in Zambia. PLoS One 2015;10(4):e0122169.
58. Zhuang Y, Yang H. The significance of nonsurgical therapies for cervical infection of high-risk human papilloma virus: A systematic review and meta-analysis. J Obstet Gynaecol Res 2023;49(9):2213–31.
59. Prudden HJ, Achilles SL, Schocken C, et al. Understanding the public health value and defining preferred product characteristics for therapeutic human papillomavirus (HPV) vaccines: World Health Organization consultations, October 2021-March 2022. Vaccine 2022;40(41):5843–55.
60. Sahasrabuddhe VV, Parham GP, Mwanahamuntu MH, et al. Cervical cancer prevention in low- and middle-income countries: feasible, affordable, essential. Cancer Prev Res (Phila) 2012;5(1):11–7.
61. Canfell K, Kim JJ, Brisson M, et al. Mortality impact of achieving WHO cervical cancer elimination targets: a comparative modelling analysis in 78 low-income and lower-middle-income countries. Lancet 2020;395(10224):591–603.

Gastrointestinal Cancer Precursor Conditions and Their Detection

Asaf Maoz, MD[a,b,1], Nicolette J. Rodriguez, MD, MPH[b,c,d,1],
Matthew B. Yurgelun, MD[a,b,2], Sapna Syngal, MD, MPH[a,2,*]

KEYWORDS

- Lynch syndrome • Polyposis • Hereditary pancreatic cancer • CDH1
- Cancer prevention • Cancer detection

KEY POINTS

- Many gastrointestinal cancers arise from detectable precursor lesions, presenting an opportunity for cancer prevention and interception.
- Hereditary cancer syndromes inform our understanding of cancer development and progression, as well as the management of cancer precursor lesions.
- Further research is needed to advance chemoprevention and immunoprevention strategies for individuals with hereditary cancer syndromes and individuals with nonhereditary cancer precursor lesions.

INTRODUCTION

Gastrointestinal (GI) cancers are a leading cause of cancer morbidity and mortality.[1] In the United States, GI cancers are predicted to lead to over 170,000 deaths in 2023 alone, accounting for 28% of cancer-related deaths.[1] Many GI cancers arise from distinct precursor lesions, presenting an opportunity for cancer prevention and interception. Hereditary cancer syndromes, in which precursor lesions are common, have informed our understanding of basic biological principles of cancer development and progression, as well as the clinical management of precursor lesions in the broader

[a] Dana-Farber Cancer Institute, 450 Brookline Avenue, Boston, MA 02215, USA; [b] Harvard Medical School, Boston, MA, USA; [c] Division of Gastroenterology, Hepatology and Endoscopy, Brigham and Women's Hospital, 75 Francis Street, Boston MA 02115, USA; [d] Division of Cancer Genetics and Prevention, 450 Brookline Avenue, Boston MA 02215, USA
[1] Co-first authors.
[2] Co-senior authors.
* Corresponding author. Dana-Farber Cancer Institute, 450 Brookline Avenue, Boston, MA 02215.
E-mail address: sapna_syngal@dfci.harvard.edu
Twitter: @asaf_maoz (A.M.); @Dr_NJRodriguez (N.J.R.); @MattYurgelun (M.B.Y.)

Hematol Oncol Clin N Am 38 (2024) 783–811
https://doi.org/10.1016/j.hoc.2024.04.002
0889-8588/24/© 2024 Elsevier Inc. All rights reserved.
hemonc.theclinics.com

population. Deleterious monogenic germline variants are thought to lead to approximately 5% to 10% of GI cancers.[2] Polygenic variation also contributes to the risk of GI cancer, including among individuals with a monogenic germline variant.[3] This review will focus on the leading causes of hereditary GI cancer, as well as the management of common precursor lesions of the GI tract.

We review hereditary predisposition to and precursor conditions of the colorectum, stomach and esophagus, and pancreas. Hereditary cancer syndromes often predispose to neoplasm in more than one organ and may be discussed later in more than one section. Hereditary neuroendocrine cancer syndromes and syndromes with insufficient evidence to guide management are outside the scope of this review.

COLORECTAL CANCER PREDISPOSITION AND PRECURSOR CONDITIONS
Lynch Syndrome

Lynch syndrome (LS) is an autosomal dominant syndrome caused by germline deleterious variants in one of the DNA mismatch repair (MMR) genes—*MLH1*, *MSH2*, *MSH6*, and *PMS2*.[4] Epigenetic silencing of *MLH1* and *MSH2* can also cause LS, the latter secondary to deletions in the *EPCAM* gene.[4] LS is the most common hereditary cause of GI cancer.[5] The population prevalence of LS and the relative frequencies of alterations in each of the MMR genes vary by population.[5–10] In the United States, LS is estimated to affect approximately 1 in 300 to 400 individuals.[5,7,8]

Within the GI tract, LS is associated with colorectal cancer (CRC), small bowel, gastric, and pancreaticobiliary cancers[11,12] (**Table 1**). The cancer risks associated with LS extend, however, beyond the GI tract and include endometrial, ovarian, urinary tract, prostate, skin, and brain cancers.[11–14] It is important to note that female individuals with LS have a cumulative risk of gynecologic cancers that is of similar or larger magnitude as the risk of colon cancer.[12]

While historically regarded as a single syndrome, there is variation in the cancer risks associated with germline alterations in each of the MMR genes (see **Table 1**), and management recommendations vary accordingly.[15,16] *MLH1*-LS and *MSH2*-LS are highly penetrant, with a lifetime cumulative risk of LS-cancer of over 70% for both male and female individuals.[12] *MSH2*-LS likely has the broadest spectrum of cancer risk, with a particularly high risk of urinary tract cancer. *EPCAM*-LS is thought to have a similar phenotype as *MSH2*-LS but data are limited. *MSH6*-LS is characterized by a higher lifetime risk of gynecologic cancers than colorectal cancer. *PMS2*-LS is the most common form of LS in the United States, leading to a lifetime risk of LS-cancers of approximately 35%. The cancer risks associated with *PMS2*-LS pertain predominantly to the colon and the endometrium.[12]

Most LS-associated cancers acquire a second, somatic, alteration in the affected MMR gene, leading to DNA MMR deficiency (MMRD) of the tumor. MMRD results in a high rate of mutations of both single nucleotide variations and insertion/deletion mutations, particularly at DNA microsatellites (termed microsatellite instability [MSI]).[4] MMR proficient tumors can also occur in individuals with LS, particularly in *MSH6*-LS and *PMS2*-LS.[17]

The precursor lesions associated with LS and their contribution to cancer risk have been studied primarily in the colon and rectum.[18] Emerging data suggest that there are several molecular pathways of CRC development in LS, underpinning distinct precursor lesions[11,12,19] (**Fig. 1**). MMRD can occur either early, before the acquisition of key driver mutations, or at a later stage in adenoma development.[18,20] Recent data suggest that early MMRD is the more common pathway.[18,21] Indeed, MMRD has been detected in nondysplastic colonic crypts, suggesting that MMRD can be a very early event,

Table 1
Lynch syndrome gastrointestinal cancer risk and management recommendations [2,15,16,41]

GI organ	MLH1		MSH2/EPCAM		MSH6		PMS2	
	Cancer risk estimate	Screening recommendations	Cancer risk estimate	Screening recommendations	Cancer risk estimate	Screening recommendations	Cancer risk estimate	Screening recommendations
Colon and rectum	46%–61%	Colonoscopy every 1–2 y, starting at age 20–25 y[a]	33%–52%	Colonoscopy every 1–2 y, starting at age 20–25 y[a]	10%–44%	Colonoscopy every 1–3 y, starting at age 30–35 y[a]	8.7%–20%	Colonoscopy every 1–3 y, starting at age 30–35 y[a]
Stomach	5%–7%	EGD every 2–4 y, starting at age 30–40 y[b]	0.2%–9.0%	EGD every 2–4 y, starting at age 30–40 y[b]	≤1%–7.9%	EGD every 2–4 y, starting at age 30–40 y[b]	Insufficient data	Consider EGD every 2–4 y, starting at age 30–40 y[b]
Small bowel	0.4%–11%	See stomach	1.1%–10%	See stomach	≤1%–4%	See stomach	0.1%–0.3%	See stomach
Pancreas	6.20%	Consider annual screening starting at age 50 y, if meeting family history criteria[c]	0.5%–1.6%	Consider annual screening starting at age 50 y, if meeting family history criteria[c]	1.4%–1.6%	Consider annual screening starting at age 50 y, if meeting family history criteria[c]	≤1% to 1.6%	Insufficient data to recommend screening[c]
Biliary tract	1.9%–3.7%	No specific recommendations	0.02%–1.7%	No specific recommendations	0.2%–≤1%	No specific recommendations	0.2% to ≤1%	No specific recommendations

[a] Or 2–5 y earlier than the earliest CRC in the family, whichever is earlier.
[b] Testing for H pylori and eradication, if positive, is recommended.
[c] Pancreatic cancer (PDAC) screening is currently to be considered in the setting of ≥1 first-degree or second-degree relative with pancreatic cancer. Screening is performed annually, alternating between MRCP and EUS. Screening should begin 10 y before the earliest PDAC in the family or at the age of 50 y, whichever is earlier.

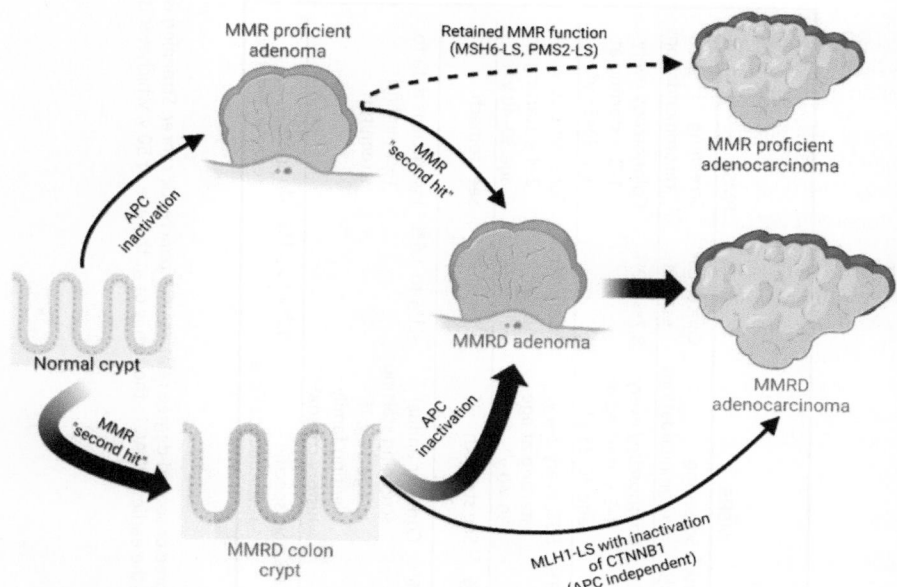

Fig. 1. LS colorectal cancer development and progression differs across MMR genes. Most LS-associated colorectal cancers are thought to arise via early acquisition of somatic MMRD, followed by progression to MMRD adenoma and carcinoma. In *MLH1*-LS, direct progression to carcinoma without an intermediate adenoma phase may occur. MMRD can also be acquired after an adenoma has developed. In a minority of cases, MMR-proficient adenomas may progress to MMR-proficient adenocarcinomas, particularly in *MSH6*-LS and *PMS2*-LS. Figure created with BioRender.com.

preceding adenoma formation.[21–23] *MSH2*, *MSH6*, and *PMS2* associated CRC is thought to develop commonly by acquisition of somatic mutations in the *APC* gene, leading to adenomatous polyp growth via activation of Wnt signaling (see "Polyposis Syndromes" section).[19,24] However, some *MLH1*-associated CRCs are hypothesized to evolve directly from colonic crypts, independent of *APC*. These tumors are thought to acquire mutations in *CTNNB1* (beta-catenin) and bypass the adenomatous polyp phase.[18,25,26] Further studies are needed to validate and refine these models of carcinogenesis in LS and determine the associated implications for colonoscopic surveillance.

Frequent colonoscopic surveillance is the mainstay of CRC early detection and prevention in LS (see **Table 1**). *MLH1*-LS and *MSH2*-LS are characterized by accelerated carcinogenesis, which is thought to develop within 2 to 3 years, in comparison with 10 or more years in sporadic CRC.[27,28] High-quality colonoscopy with polypectomy at frequent intervals reduces the incidence of CRC in individuals with LS.[29] There are limited data regarding the outcomes of upper GI endoscopic surveillance and pancreatic cancer screening among individuals with LS.[30–32] Screening recommendations are discussed in **Table 1** and under "Pancreatic cancer predisposition and precursor conditions".

Beyond the prevention afforded by colonoscopies, high-quality data support the use of aspirin for the prevention of colorectal cancer among individuals with LS.[33,34] The randomized CAPP2 trial demonstrated a reduction in colorectal cancer incidence for individuals with LS who were randomized to aspirin treatment versus placebo (9% vs 13%, HR = 0.65).[33] The CAPP3 trial is ongoing with the goal of determining if lower doses of aspirin are equally effective for chemoprevention in LS (NCT02497820). Recent data suggest that resistant starch, also studied in the CAPP2 trial, may be beneficial for the prevention of upper GI cancers in LS.[35] The mechanisms driving the preventative effects of aspirin and resistance starch in individuals with LS have not been definitively established.

Immunoprevention is actively being explored for individuals with LS. As discussed above, MMRD leads to a high somatic mutational burden in LS-associated cancers. Neoantigens that arise from MMRD are thought to elicit an immune reaction that can restrict cancer growth or lead to cancer regression, both spontaneously and in response to T-cell immune checkpoint inhibitors.[36–38] While immune checkpoint inhibitors are effective for treating established LS-associated cancers with MMRD, it is unclear if they offer a preventative benefit. A study of patients with LS who received immunotherapy for an established malignancy suggests a persistent risk of precursor lesions and malignancy.[39] Cancer vaccines for the prevention of LS-associated cancers are also in clinical development.[40] These include vaccines that target tumor-associated antigens that are not specific to LS (NCT05419011), as well as LS-specific vaccines that target neoantigens that arise as a result of MMRD (NCT05078866).

Polyposis Syndromes

Multiple hereditary cancer syndromes result in polyposis of the GI tract,[41,42] most involving the colon and rectum. Polyposis syndromes vary clinically in their inheritance pattern, molecular etiology, polyp type and burden, and extracolonic manifestations (**Table 2**).

Familial adenomatous polyposis (FAP) is the most common hereditary polyposis syndrome of the GI tract. FAP is an autosomal dominant syndrome caused by pathogenic germline variants in the *APC* gene. Classic FAP is highly penetrant, leading to hundreds to thousands of adenomatous polyps in the colon and rectum, and a lifetime CRC risk of virtually 100%. Attenuated FAP is clinically distinguished from classic FAP as a syndrome with less than 100 colonic polyps; it is associated with germline alterations in the 3′ or 5′ portion of the *APC* gene.[43] Individuals with FAP often have polyposis of the upper GI tract, as well, leading to cancers of the stomach, small bowel, and ampulla of Vater.[44–47] Additional tumors associated with FAP include desmoid tumors, thyroid cancer, hepatoblastoma, and medulloblastoma.[48–50]

CRC carcinogenesis in FAP is driven by a somatic second hit in the *APC* gene.[51,52] This in turn leads to unopposed β-catenin activity, activating the Wnt signaling pathway, as well as chromosomal instability.[24] Germline alterations in *RNF43* and *AXIN2* also lead to polyposis via the Wnt signaling pathway, though they cause phenotypically distinct syndromes from FAP.[53] Acquired somatic mutations in additional oncogenes (eg, *KRAS*) or tumor suppressor genes (eg, *TP53*) are thought to drive tumorigenesis, in a process similar to the sporadic adenoma to carcinoma process.[54,55] Spatially separated tumors can originate from the same cancer-primed cell in patients with FAP, indicating that somatic alterations may occur in a macroscopically normal epithelium, before the appearance of clinically identifiable adenomas.[56] Multiple other mechanisms of polyposis exist, including alterations in kinase and phosphatase activity, DNA base excision repair, DNA polymerase activity, TGF-β signaling, and others (see **Table 2**).

Esophagogastroduodenoscopy (EGD) and colonoscopy are the mainstay of cancer early detection for individuals with polyposis syndromes (see "Management of precursor lesions" below). Small bowel visualization with video capsule endoscopy or CT/MRI enterography is recommended for syndromes with a high risk of small bowel cancer (see **Table 2**). In polyposis syndromes with a low to moderate polyp burden,

Table 2
Polyposis syndromes of the gastrointestinal tract [2,15,41,42]

Polyposis Syndrome	Gene(s)	Molecular Pathway	Colonic Polyposis Phenotype	Colon Cancer Risk	Colon Cancer Risk management[a]	Extracolonic GI Polyposis/Cancer Risk and management[a]	Extra-GI Cancer Risk
Classic FAP	APC	Wnt signaling	≥100 adenomas	100%	Colectomy with ileorectal anastomosis, or total proctocolectomy with ileal pouch-anal anastomosis, or proctocolectomy with end ileostomy. When applicable, the remaining bowel should undergo endoscopic surveillance every 6–12 mo	Gastric, duodenal, and ampullary cancer: EGD including complete visualization of the ampulla of Vater at age 20–25 y or earlier based on family history, with further intervals dependent on findings. Pancreatic cancer: no specific screening recommendations	Intra-abdominal desmoid tumors, thyroid cancer, hepatoblastoma, medulloblastoma, and other central nervous system (CNS) cancers
Attenuated FAP	APC	Wnt signaling	10–<100 adenomas	70%	Colonoscopy every 1–2 y. Surgical approaches as in classic FAP may be warranted depending on phenotype	Gastric, duodenal, and ampullary cancer: EGD including complete visualization of the ampulla of Vater at age 20–25 y or earlier based on family history, with further intervals dependent on findings	Thyroid cancer

GAPPS	APC	Wnt signaling	No polyposis	Insufficient data	Colonoscopy at time of diagnosis to exclude colon polyposis	Stomach fundic gland polyposis and cancer risk: annual gastroscopy from age 15 y. Consider risk-reducing total gastrectomy from third decade. Pancreatic cancer: no specific screening recommendations	No definitive risk
MAP	Biallelic MUTYH (AR)	DNA base excision repair	10–100; adenomas and hyperplastic polyps > serrated, sessile serrated, mixed polyps	70%–90%	Colonoscopy every 1–2 y. Surgical approaches as in classic FAP may be warranted for an adenoma burden that cannot be handled endoscopically	Gastric, duodenal and ampullary cancer: EGD including complete visualization of the ampulla of Vater at age 20–25 y or earlier based on family history, with further intervals dependent on findings	No definitive risk
Juvenile polyposis	SMAD4, BMPR1A	TGF-β/BMP signaling	≥5 Hamartomatous/ juvenile polyps	50%	Colonoscopy starting at 12–15 y. If polyps are found, repeat every 2–3 y or sooner based on findings. If no polyps, then resume at 18 y every 1–3 y	Stomach cancer: EGD starting at 12–15 y. If polyps are found, repeat every 2–3 y or earlier based on findings. If no polyps, then resume at 18 y every 1–3 y	No definitive risk

(continued on next page)

Table 2
(continued)

Polyposis Syndrome	Gene(s)	Molecular Pathway	Colonic Polyposis Phenotype	Colon Cancer Risk	Colon Cancer Risk management[a]	Extracolonic GI Polyposis/Cancer Risk and management[a]	Extra-GI Cancer Risk
Polymerase proofreading associated polyposis	POLD, POLE	DNA proofreading and replication	30 – >100 adenomas	>20%	Colonoscopy at 25–30 y and repeat every 2–3 y if negative. If polyps are found, colonoscopy every 1–2 y	Insufficient data	Insufficient data
Peutz-Jeghers	STK11 (LKB1)	Serine/threonine protein kinase activity	≥2 Peutz-Jeghers-type hamartomatous polyps	39%	Colonoscopy starting at 8–10 y. If polyps are found, repeat every 2–3 y. If no polyps, then resume at age 18 y	Stomach and small intestine cancer: EGD at intervals as colonoscopy. Small bowel visualization (video capsule endoscopy or CT/MRI enterography) at baseline with follow-up interval based on findings, but at least by age 18 y, then every 2–3 y. Pancreatic cancer: MRCP/EUS annually, starting at 30–35 y or 10 y earlier than the earliest diagnosis in the family	Breast, endometrial, cervical, lung, ovarian, and testes

Syndrome	Gene	Function/Pathway	Polyps	CRC risk	Surveillance	Other risk	Associated cancers
PTEN hamartoma tumor syndrome	PTEN	Phosphatase activity, PI3K/AKT	0 – >100; mixed polyposis: hamartomas, hyperplastic, adenomas, inflammatory, ganglioneuromas	11%–20%	Colonoscopy, starting at age 35 y unless symptomatic or if close relative with CRC before age 40 y, then start 5–10 y before the earliest known CRC in the family. Colonoscopy should be done every 5 y	No definitive risk	Breast, thyroid, endometrial, kidney cancer, and melanoma
NTHL1 tumor syndrome	Biallelic NTHL1 (AR)	DNA base excision repair	1–100; adenomas > serrated, sessile serrated, hyperplastic polyps	>20%	Colonoscopy at age 25–30 y and repeat every 2–3 y if negative. If polyps are found, colonoscopy every 1–2 y	Duodenal cancer: insufficient data	Breast, endometrial, urothelial carcinomas, hematologic malignancies, squamous cell carcinoma of the head, neck, and cervix
Serrated polyposis syndrome	RNF43, (MUTYH)	Wnt signaling, (DNA base excision repair)	5 – >100; serrated lesions/polyps (hyperplastic polyp, sessile serrated lesion without or with dysplasia, traditional serrated adenoma, and unclassified serrated adenoma)	Insufficient data	Colonoscopy until all polyps ≥5 mm are removed, then colonoscopy every 1–3 y depending on findings	Insufficient data	Insufficient data

(continued on next page)

Table 2
(continued)

Polyposis Syndrome	Gene(s)	Molecular Pathway	Colonic Polyposis Phenotype	Colon Cancer Risk	Colon Cancer Risk management[a]	Extracolonic GI Polyposis/Cancer Risk and management[a]	Extra-GI Cancer Risk
Hereditary mixed polyposis syndrome	GREM1	TGF-β/BMP signaling	Mixed polyposis; adenomas and a unique polyp composed of a mixture of hyperplastic polyp and inflammatory polyp–type changes are the most frequent	11%–20%	Colonoscopy at age 25–30 y and repeat every 2–3 y if negative. If polyps are found, colonoscopy every 1–2 y	Insufficient data	Insufficient data
Constitutional MMR deficiency	Biallelic PMS2, MSH6, MLH1, MSH2 (AR)	DNA MMR	0 - > 100	Insufficient data	Annual colonoscopy starting at age 6 y. Once polyps are identified, repeat every 6 mo	Small intestine polyposis and cancer: EGD and video capsule endoscopy starting at 8 y	Hematologic, CNS, sarcomas, and genitourinary
AXIN2	AXIN2	Wnt signaling	0 – >100, mainly adenomas	Insufficient data	Colonoscopy at age 25–30 y and repeat every 2–3 y if negative. If polyps are found, colonoscopy every 1–2 y	Insufficient data	Insufficient data
MBD4-associated neoplasia syndrome	Biallelic MBD4 (AR)	DNA base excision repair	15–100+ adenomas	Insufficient data	Colonoscopy at age 18–20 y or date of diagnosis and repeat every 2–3 y if negative	Insufficient data	Acute myeloid leukemia, uveal melanoma

| MSH3-associated polyposis syndrome | Biallelic MSH3 (AR) | DNA mismatch repair | 30 – >100 adenomas | Insufficient data | Colonoscopy at age 25–30 y and repeat every 2–3 y if negative. If polyps are found, colonoscopy every 1–2 y | Insufficient data | Insufficient data |
| MLH3-associated polyposis syndrome | Biallelic MLH3 (AR) | DNA MMR | 30 – >100 adenomas | Insufficient data | Begin high-quality colonoscopy at age 25–30 y and repeat every 2–3 y if negative. If polyps are found, colonoscopy every 1–2 y | Insufficient data | Insufficient data |

[a] Surgical resection should be considered for high-risk lesions or when polyps cannot be managed endoscopically in the colon, stomach, and small bowel. AR, autosomal recessive.

endoscopic management serves as the primary prevention strategy. However, when endoscopic management is not feasible because of a high polyp burden, prophylactic surgery, including colectomy/proctocolectomy, pancreaticoduodenectomy, and/or gastrectomy, may be considered.

Chemoprevention and chemointerception trials have been conducted almost exclusively for FAP. Sulindac and other NSAIDs have been evaluated in several trials as monotherapy or in combination with other agents.[57,58] The combination of the NSAID sulindac and the EGFR inhibitor erlotinib has been shown to reduce colorectal and duodenal polyp burden in FAP over short-term follow-up.[59,60] An irreversible inhibitor of ornithine decarboxylase, eflornithine, has been suggested to have a role in the prevention of colonic disease progression in FAP, but further studies are needed to confirm these findings.[61] Despite demonstrating a reduction of polyp burden, these regimens have not been definitively shown to alter clinical management for individuals with FAP and have not received Food and Drug Administration approval for this indication.

Management of precursor lesions

Colorectal polyps. CRC screening is recommended for all asymptomatic adults aged 45 years or older who are at an average risk of CRC.[62,63] The recommended age to initiate screening was changed from 50 to 45 years in recent years because of an increasing incidence of young-onset CRC. The causes of this increase in CRC incidence are poorly understood, but they have been largely attributed to lifestyle and environmental factors, as this increased risk is associated with a birth-cohort effect. Individuals born around 1990 have up to 4 times the risk of rectal cancer and twice the risk of colon cancer of individuals born around 1950.[64–66] Various screening strategies are now recommended for individuals at average risk for CRC, including stool-based tests, CT colonography, sigmoidoscopy, and colonoscopy.[63]

Colonoscopy is performed in the setting of routine colon cancer screening, but also as follow-up of abnormal CRC screening tests, surveillance postpolypectomy or CRC resection/treatment, or for diagnostic purposes.[67] Colonoscopy can prevent CRC through the disruption of precursor lesions, such as polyps, including tubular adenomas and sessile serrated polyps (SSPs).[68] The sensitivity of stool-based and blood-based tests for precursor lesions is limited,[62,69,70] and positive findings require follow-up with a colonoscopy. The development of these polypoid lesions and CRC occurs through 3 distinct pathways, the chromosomal instability, the MSI, and the CpG island methylator phenotype.

Risk factors for the development of traditional adenomas and SSPs include smoking, obesity, and heavy alcohol use.[71] Physical activity and the use of aspirin is associated with a lower risk of developing adenomas and an advanced adenoma or large SSP, respectively. These risk factors largely mirror risk factors for CRC development,[71] although the association of aspirin use with a decreased risk of CRC has been called into question.[72] The presence of one or more of these risk factors does not typically alter CRC surveillance recommendations.[63] Apart from the hereditary syndromes discussed earlier, there are additional personal and familial risk factors that warrant specialized surveillance, the specifics of which are outside the scope of this review. These include a personal history of inflammatory bowel disease, cystic fibrosis, and childhood cancer treated with chemotherapy or abdominal radiation therapy and a family history of CRC without a detectable pathogenic germline variant.[73–77]

Individuals with precancerous colorectal polyps have a higher risk for colorectal cancer compared to the general population and thus interval surveillance colonoscopy will be based on age, personal history, genetic susceptibility, family history, procedural findings, prep quality, examination quality, and comorbidities.[67]

Overall, individuals that are found to have an adenoma at baseline colonoscopy, have a 1.3 fold risk of developing CRC compared to the general population.[78] Adenomas can be risk stratified as a low-risk adenoma (<10 mm in size), advanced adenoma (≥10 mm in size, tubulovillous or villous histology, high-grade dysplasia), advanced neoplasia (advanced adenoma or CRC), or high-risk adenoma (advanced neoplasia or ≥3 adenomas).[67] Patients who are found to have an advanced adenoma compared to a non-advanced adenoma have a higher risk of developing CRC compared to the general population (Standardized incidence ratios of 2.23 and 0.68, respectively).[78] Patients undergoing routine recommended surveillance colonoscopy for an advanced adenoma have a 2.05% 10-year cumulative risk of developing CRC.[78] Furthermore, among patients found to have an SSP or SSP with dysplasia compared to no polyps, the odds of developing CRC are 3 fold and 5 fold, respectively.[79]

Risk-stratification as well as timing of surveillance colonoscopy after baseline colonoscopy for both adenomas and SSPs are based on number of polyps, size of polyps, and histology (**Fig. 2**). These recommendations have been previously summarized and well described.[67]

Importantly, the recommended interval for the second-surveillance colonoscopy among postpolypectomy patients is based on the risk-stratification of findings identified on baseline and first-surveillance colonoscopies.[67] Overall, colonoscopy provides the opportunity to remove precursor CRC lesions and to intercept CRC early when it is more amenable to treatment and surgical options.

GASTROESOPHAGEAL CANCER PREDISPOSITION AND PRECURSOR CONDITIONS
Hereditary Syndromes

Several hereditary cancer syndromes predispose to gastric cancer (**Table 3**). The prevalence of any germline alteration in cancer predisposition genes among patients with gastric cancer is in the range of 10%,[80–82] but causality has only been established

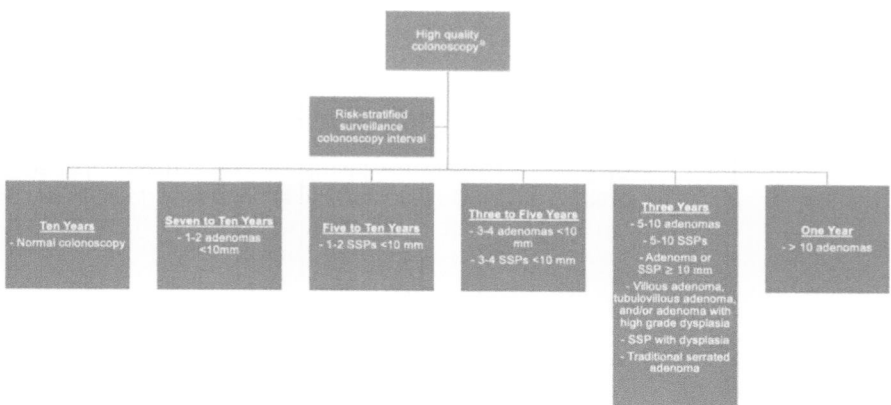

Fig. 2. Recommendations for timing of surveillance colonoscopy after polypectomy of an adenoma or SSP. [a]High quality colonoscopy as defined by the 2020 US Multi-Society Task Force on Colorectal Cancer (*Adapted with permission from* Elsevier: Gupta S, Lieberman D, Anderson JC, et al. Recommendations for Follow-Up After Colonoscopy and Polypectomy: A Consensus Update by the US Multi-Society Task Force on Colorectal Cancer. Gastrointest Endosc. 2020;91(3):463-485.e5. https://doi.org/10.1016/j.gie.2020.01.014. Please refer to the US Multi-Society Task Force on Colorectal Cancer for additional recommendations on follow-up colonoscopy for hyperplastic polyps.)

Table 3
Hereditary cancer syndromes predisposing to gastric cancer [2,85,93]

Gene/s	Gastric Cancer Risk	Gastric Cancer Risk management[a]	Other Cancer Risks
CDH1	33%–42%	Prophylactic total gastrectomy at age 18–40 y, or earlier if there is a family history of gastric cancer at an age <25 y. Individuals who elect not to undergo prophylactic gastrectomy should be offered screening every 6–12 mo by upper endoscopy with multiple random biopsies	Lobular breast cancer
CTNNA1	49%–57%	Insufficient data to guide management. Consider management similar to CDH1	Insufficient data
Lynch syndrome (MLH1, MSH2/EPCAM, MSH6, PMS2)	See **Table 1**	See **Table 1**	See **Table 1**
Juvenile polyposis syndrome (SMAD4)	21%	See **Table 2**	See **Table 2**
Peutz-Jeghers syndrome (STK11)	29%	See **Table 2**	See **Table 2**
FAP (APC)	2%	See **Table 2**	See **Table 2**
Li-Fraumeni syndrome (TP53)	10.7%	EGD every 2–5 y starting at age 25 y	See **Table 4**
BRCA2, ATM, PALB2, BRCA1	Insufficient data	Insufficient data to guide management	See **Table 4**

[a] Testing for *H pylori* and eradication if positive can be considered regardless of recommendations for endoscopic surveillance or surgery.

for a limited number of genes. Overall, it is estimated that 3% to 5% of gastric cancers can be attributed to monogenic hereditary cancer syndromes.

Hereditary diffuse gastric cancer (HDGC) is a gastric-cancer predominant syndrome.[83,84] HDGC is caused by germline deleterious alterations in *CDH1*, encoding the E-cadherin gene, a major component of the adherens junction of epithelial cells.[85] HDGC is associated with diffuse type gastric cancer with signet ring cell morphology, as well as lobular breast cancer. The cancer risk associated with HDGC is still being refined. Initial estimates were likely inflated because of ascertainment bias; a large proportion of families with germline alterations in *CDH1* do not meet clinical criteria for HDGC and are found incidentally.[86–88] Germline alterations in *CTNNA1* also predispose to diffuse gastric cancer,[83,84,89,90] but the risk of lobular breast cancer has not been established.[91] *CTNNA1* encodes the alpha-catenin protein, also an adherens junction protein.[92]

The precursor lesions of HDGC are microscopic signet-ring cell foci. These include lesions replacing the normal gland cells (in situ signet-ring cell carcinoma) or pagetoid spread of signet-ring cells below the preserved epithelium.[85] In approximately 95% of cases of HDGC associated with *CDH1* germline alterations, foci of signet-ring cells are detected in the lamina propria (stage T1a). The discrepancy between the near-ubiquitous finding of T1a lesions and the partial penetrance of diffuse gastric cancer suggests that many T1a lesions have indolent behavior and do not progress rapidly to advanced cancer. The recommended management for individuals with HDGC has been to consider a prophylactic total gastrectomy at an early age (see **Table 3**), before invasive cancer develops.[85,93] Specialized endoscopic surveillance protocols, which include multiple biopsies, have been proposed as a method of cancer interception for individuals who do not undergo prophylactic gastrectomy.[94–96] Accumulating experience from the implementation of such protocols suggests that endoscopic surveillance may be an alternative to surgery in individuals with *CDH1* alterations who decline total gastrectomy. However, predictors of progression are not well defined, and there are no sufficiently reliable methods to detect progression when it occurs.

There are no established nonoperative interventions to prevent gastric cancer in HDGC. As a presumed modifiable risk factor, *Helicobacter pylori* detection and eradication are recommended,[85] and this recommendation extends to other hereditary cancer syndromes that may predispose to gastric cancer, such as LS.

Hereditary predisposition to esophageal cancer is less well characterized. Rare syndromes that predispose to *squamous cell* carcinoma of the esophagus have been described, including Tylosis with esophageal cancer,[97–99] Bloom syndrome,[100] and Fanconi anemia.[101] Screening recommendations are based on limited data but include consideration of an upper endoscopy starting at early adulthood.[102] Hereditary predisposition to esophageal *adenocarcinoma* (EAC) is less well understood, and there is no consensus regarding specific screening recommendations. There is notable overlap between the genes proposed to predispose to EAC and gastric adenocarcinoma. Recent data suggest that pathogenic variants in *ATM* and *TP53* predispose to EAC, as well as to progression from its precursor lesion, Barret's esophagus (BE), to adenocarcinoma.[103] Genes involved in the DNA homologous recombination pathway (eg, *BRCA1/2*) have also been suggested to predispose to gastroesophageal cancer[80–82,103] but causality has not been definitively established.

Management of Precursor Lesions

Gastric intestinal metaplasia

Gastric intestinal metaplasia (GIM) is a precursor lesion for gastric adenocarcinoma as it may develop into dysplasia, which may progress to gastric cancer.[104] GIM can be further characterized by histologic subtype as incomplete (has some colonic type intestinal metaplasia [IM]) versus complete (small intestinal type IM) and anatomic location as extensive (involves the gastric body and either the antrum and/or incisura) versus limited (only involves the gastric antrum and/or incisura). Individuals with incomplete and/or extensive GIM have the highest risk of progressing to gastric cancer.[105] Higher risk patients with GIM include individuals with incomplete and/or extensive GIM or individuals with a family history of gastric cancer. In addition, patients at an overall increased risk for gastric cancer, include individuals who immigrated from high gastric cancer incidence regions and individuals from historically marginalized racial/ethnic backgrounds.[105]

Among patients who have had gastric biopsies, the prevalence of GIM is approximately 4.8%.[106] At 5 year follow-up, the cumulative incidence of gastric cancer among individuals with GIM is 1.1% and 1.6% at 10 years.[107] Importantly, this prevalence and incidence data were drawn from studies conducted in North America, South America, Europe and Asia, where population risk differs across regions.[107]

In Asian countries, particularly Eastern Asia, there is a higher incidence and mortality rate associated with gastric cancer, with some risk factors including higher rates of *H pylori* infection, diet, and hereditary predisposition, as mentioned above.[108] As a result, some countries in that region have implemented national screening guidelines that are associated with reductions in gastric cancer mortality.[109]

However, the United States is considered a low-incidence country with 26,500 gastric cancer cases diagnosed in 2023, with the most common location of gastric cancer being noncardia gastric cancers.[110] As a result, population-based screening initiatives have not been implemented. However, incidentally identified GIM on endoscopic biopsies has led to the development of practice guidelines on how to best manage these findings routinely.[105]

Eradication of *H pylori* with eradication confirmation is recommended for patients with GIM and *H pylori*.[105] Among patients with incidentally identified GIM, endoscopic surveillance every 3 to 5 years with random biopsies of the gastric body and antrum as well as targeted biopsies of any concerning lesions, can be considered based on informed discussions regarding the risks/benefits of the procedure as a reduction in gastric cancer mortality has not yet been delineated.[105]

Lastly, guidelines also do not recommend short-interval endoscopy to risk stratify patients with incidentally identified GIM. However, based on informed clinical discussions, patients who are at higher risk, as delineated earlier, or patients who had any high-risk lesions or concerns regarding the thoroughness of their initial endoscopic evaluation can undergo a repeat upper endoscopy in 1 year for further risk stratification (ie, anatomic extent and histologic subtype).[105]

Barrett's esophagus

BE describes the replacement of normal esophageal squamous epithelium by metaplastic columnar epithelium with goblet cells.[111] This metaplastic mucosal change in the distal esophagus is also denoted as IM and is associated with chronic gastroesophageal reflux disease (GERD).[112] Approximately 5% to 12% of patients with chronic GERD develop BE.[113,114] BE is considered the precursor lesion for EAC with histologic progression from BE with no dysplasia to low-grade dysplasia, high-grade dysplasia, and ultimately EAC.[115]

As BE can be a clinically silent disease, prevalence estimates are predominately based upon patient populations that present for endoscopic evaluation in the setting of GERD symptoms. In the United States, the prevalence of BE is estimated to be 5.6%, with other estimates ranging from 0.4 to greater than 20% in the general population based on the population studied and diagnosis study criteria.[116–120] Compared to the general population, individuals with BE have a 10 fold to 55 fold risk of developing EAC.[121] Among individuals with high-grade dysplasia (HGD) specifically, the incidence of developing EAC within the first 7 years of diagnosis is 6.58 per 100 patient-years.[122]

Risk factors for BE include age over 50 years, central obesity, tobacco use, and family history.[112] In addition, White race and male sex are risk factors for BE with BE being more common in White and male populations and uncommon in Black, Asian/Pacific Islander, and female populations.[112,123] As a result, the American College of Gastroenterology recommends screening endoscopy for individuals with chronic GERD symptoms and 3 or more of the risk factors delineated above including a family history of BE or EAC in one or more first-degree relatives.[124] The American Gastroenterological Association has similar recommendations.[125]

Endoscopic suspicion of BE requires that columnar epithelium be identified at least 1 cm or more proximal to the gastroesophageal junction.[112] When BE is suspected on initial white-light endoscopy, this mucosal change is characterized by a salmon-colored mucosa.[112] Once suspected, at least 8 endoscopic biopsies are recommended to identify the presence of IM.[112] The Seattle Biopsy Sampling Protocol is recommended by multiple societies and targeted biopsies of any identified mucosal abnormalities are also indicated.[112,126] If IM is not identified, a repeat endoscopy with biopsies is recommended in 1 to 2 years.[112] However, if IM is identified, this mucosal change is further stratified into BE with no dysplasia, BE with indefinite dysplasia (IND), and BE with low-grade dysplasia (LGD), HGD, or early EAC.[112] If dysplasia or EAC is suspected, pathologic confirmation by a second pathologist with GI expertise is recommended for appropriate risk-stratification.[112,127]

The surveillance interval for BE with no dysplasia is based on the length of the BE segment. Among individuals with a BE segment of less than 3 cm, a repeat surveillance endoscopy is recommended in 5 years.[112] Among individuals with a BE segment of 3 cm or greater, a repeat endoscopy is recommended in 3 years.[112] In patients found to have BE with IND, treatment with a twice daily proton pump inhibitor and a repeat endoscopy within 6 months is recommended.[112]

Surveillance and management of individuals found to have LGD, HGD, intramucosal carcinoma (T1a), or submucosal cancer (T1b) are well described and briefly summarized here.[68,82] For individuals found to have LGD, an informed discussion regarding the risks and benefits of surveillance versus endoscopic eradication therapy (EET) is recommended.[112] Among patients who proceed with EET the primary endpoint is complete eradication of IM (CEIM), with ongoing surveillance endoscopy at specified intervals thereafter.[112] Among patients with HGD or intramucosal carcinoma (T1a), EET with a goal of CEIM is recommended followed by ongoing surveillance endoscopy also at specified intervals thereafter.[112,127]

Importantly, among patients with BE, chemoprophylaxis with proton pump inhibitor therapy can reduce the progression to EAC and remains an integral part of clinical management.[128]

PANCREATIC CANCER PREDISPOSITION AND PRECURSOR CONDITIONS
Hereditary Syndromes

Several distinct syndromes predispose to hereditary pancreatic cancer (HPC), including alterations in the DNA double-strand break repair pathway (specifically in the *ATM*, *BRCA2*, *BRCA1*, and *PALB2* genes), Lynch syndrome, Li-Fraumeni syndrome, and others (**Table 4**). Taken together, these syndromes account for approximately 10% of

Table 4
Hereditary pancreatic cancer syndromes[2,132,133]

Gene	PDAC Risk	Additional Criteria Suggested for PDAC Screening eligibility[a]	Age of Initiating PDAC screening[b]	Extrapancreatic GI Cancer Risk	Extra-GI Cancer Risk
STK11	32%–54%	No additional criteria	30–35	See Table 2	See Table 2
CDKN2A	>15%	No additional criteria	40	Insufficient data	Melanoma; limited data suggests sarcoma, nerve sheath tumors, and other cancers
ATM	5%–10%	Family history	50	Possibly gastric and colon cancer	Breast, prostate, and ovarian
BRCA2	5%–10%	Family history	50	Possibly gastric	Breast (female and male), ovarian, prostate, and possibly melanoma
BRCA1	<5%	Family history	50	Possibly gastric	Breast (female and male), ovarian, prostate, and possibly melanoma
PALB2	2%–10%	Family history	50	Possibly gastric	Breast (female and male), ovarian, prostate, and possibly melanoma
TP53	7.30%	Family history	50	Colorectal, gastric	Breast, sarcoma, CNS, leukemia, adrenocorticoid carcinoma, lung, thyroid, and others
MLH1	See Table 1	Family history	50	See Table 1	Uterine, ovarian, skin, urothelial, CNS, and prostate
MSH2/EPCAM	See Table 1	Family history	50	See Table 1	Uterine, ovarian, skin, urothelial, CNS, prostate, and others
MSH6	See Table 1	Family history	50	See Table 1	Uterine, ovarian, skin, urothelial, CNS, and prostate
PRSS1, SPINK1	Insufficient data	Clinical hereditary pancreatitis	40 or 20 y after onset of pancreatitis	Insufficient data	Insufficient data

[a] Family history is defined as ≥ 1 first-degree or second-degree relative with pancreatic cancer.
[b] Or 10 y younger than the earliest PDAC diagnosis in the family.

pancreatic adenocarcinoma (PDAC) cases.[129–131] The lifetime risk of PDAC differs significantly depending on the affected gene, with a particularly high risk with germline alterations in *STK11* and *CDKN2A*. There are insufficient data regarding PDAC risk modifiers among individuals with HPC; family history is used in clinical practice to guide screening recommendations.[132,133]

The precursor lesions of PDAC include pancreatic intraepithelial neoplasia (PanIN) and intraductal papillary mucinous neoplasm (IPMN).[134,135] PanIN is a microscopic lesion that is thought to be the precursor lesion for most PDACs. PanINs can be classified based on their histologic appearance as low grade and high grade; the latter is considered carcinoma in situ. The progression from PanIN to PDAC is thought to occur via sequential acquisition of somatic alterations in key oncogenes (*KRAS*) and tumor suppressor genes (*CDKN2A*, *TP53*, and *SMAD4*). *KRAS* alterations are thought to represent the earliest somatic driver, with over 90% of PDAC harboring a somatic *KRAS* alteration. IPMNs are macroscopic cystic lesions arising from the pancreatic ductal system (see "Management of Precursor Lesions" section for additional details). IPMNs are thought to harbor somatic alterations similar to PDAC but an enrichment of alterations in *GNAS* and *RNF43* in IPMNs has been described.[136] PanIN and IPMN can co-occur.[137] Mucinous cystic neoplasms (MCNs) can also progress to pancreatic cancer; MCNs are less common than IPMNs.[138]

Accumulating data from clinical trials demonstrate that screening for PDAC among individuals with HPC can detect PDAC at earlier stages. Correspondingly, screen-detected PDAC is associated with dramatically improved long-term survival.[137,139,140] Screening is associated with a high rate of detection of pancreatic cysts that require further imaging or biopsies,[141,142] as well as a less than 5% chance of undergoing surgery that is of low yield or deemed not necessary after review of final pathology.[143,144] Current screening criteria and methods are presented in **Table 4**. There is no high-quality data regarding PDAC prevention among individuals with HPC, but vaccines targeting common somatic *KRAS* alterations are being developed.[145]

Management of Precursor Lesions

Intraductal papillary mucinous neoplasms

Pancreatic IPMNs are mucinous cystic lesions that are a precursor for PDAC. IPMNs may progress from a benign IPMN to IPMN with LGD, IPMN with HGD, and invasive carcinoma.[146] These mucinous neoplasms are characterized based on the location of pancreatic duct involvement as a main duct IPMN (MD-IPMN), branch duct IPMN (BD-IPMN), or mixed type IPMN. It is difficult to discern the incidence of IPMNs, as individuals may be asymptomatic and/or have very small lesions. Previous studies assessing the prevalence of pancreatic cystic lesions that were found incidentally on cross-sectional abdominal imaging, found a prevalence ranging from 2.6% to 13.5% and a mean cyst diameter from 7.4 to 8.9 mm.[147,148]

Among those diagnosed with an IPMN, the median age at time of diagnosis is 66 to 67 years with BD-IPMNs being more commonly an incidental finding compared to MD-IPMNs or mixed-duct IPMNs.[149] In addition, most individuals with IPMNs do not have a family history of PDAC.[149] Despite this, patients with MD-IPMN or mixed-type IPMN have a 57% to 92% risk of developing an IPMN-associated carcinoma whereas patients with BD-IPMN have a 6% to 46% risk.[149,150]

Given the malignant potential of IPMNs, there are various national and international guidelines highlighting management considerations including surveillance and surgical recommendations for pancreatic cysts.[150–153] The most recently published Kyoto guidelines focus specifically on IPMNs and will be discussed in more detail. The Kyoto guidelines recommend considering surgery among individuals found to have "high-risk stigmata" of HGD or malignancy. These high-risk features include main pancreatic duct (MPD) of 10 mm or greater, an enhancing mural nodule of 5 mm or greater, obstructive jaundice in an individual with a pancreatic head cystic lesion, or patients with suspicious or positive cytology.[154] Worrisome features prompting additional evaluation can be subdivided as clinical (acute pancreatitis, elevated CA 19-9, newly diagnosed or acutely exacerbated diabetes in the last year) or imaging features (cyst ≥3 cm, enhancing mural nodule <5 mm, thickened/enhancing cystic walls, MPD 5–9 mm, abrupt change in pancreatic duct caliber with distal pancreatic atrophy, lymphadenopathy, cystic growth rate of ≥2.5 mm/12 mo).[154] Subsequent potential surgical evaluation versus surveillance is based on patient symptoms, including repeated bouts of acute pancreatitis, the presence of more than one worrisome feature, surgical candidacy and cystic size. Surveillance intervals with multidetector computed tomography, magnetic resonance cholangiopancreatography (MRCP) and/or endoscopic ultrasound (EUS) are based on the largest cyst size.[154] Overall, other guidelines, also provide surgical, endoscopic, or imaging recommendations based on risk stratification and IPMN size criteria.[151,153]

However, the Kyoto guidelines are not specifically designed for high-risk individuals, who have a personal or familial/genetic risk for PDAC. The Cancer of the Pancreas Screening Studies Consortium has released a consensus statement on the management of pancreatic cysts in high-risk populations.[137] As a result, it is imperative to interpret cystic guidelines within the context of the populations they are targeted for.

SUMMARY

Hereditary cancer syndromes of the GI tract result in a wide variety of precursor lesions and biological processes of cancer development and progression. Individuals with hereditary predisposition to cancer are ideal candidates for efforts aimed at improving early detection, such as those leveraging blood-based cancer detection. Similarly, cancer surveillance and interception are suited for individuals with nonhereditary precursor lesions. Further clinical and preclinical research is needed to inform future studies in these fields.

CLINICS CARE POINTS

- Hereditary cancer syndromes predispose to a variety of GI malignancies and precursor lesions. Screening, surveillance, and management recommendations differ based on the gene in which a germline pathogenic variant is identified, as well as clinical factors.

- LS is the most common GI cancer hereditary syndrome. LS increases the risk of malignancy in multiple GI organs, requiring multimodality surveillance, often at an early age. LS-specific cancer prevention with aspirin and resistant starch has been shown to be effective.

- Predisposition to gastric cancer is particularly high in HDGC syndrome. Prophylactic gastrectomy should be considered in young adulthood.

- The most common hereditary cancer syndromes, including LS and BRCA1/2-associated hereditary breast and ovarian cancers, also predispose to pancreatic cancer. Pancreatic cancer surveillance can detect cancer at earlier stages, leading to favorable long-term outcomes, but these encouraging results have only been demonstrated for high-risk populations undergoing screening at specialized centers.

- Multiple hereditary syndromes lead to colonic polyposis, with varying malignancy risk of extracolonic and extra-GI tract organs.

- Precursor lesions of the GI tract, including colorectal polyps, BE, GIM, and IPMNS, can occur in the absence of a diagnosed hereditary cancer syndrome, and warrant specialized surveillance and management.

DISCLOSURE

Maoz has no disclosures related to this article. N.J. Rodriguez has no disclosures related to this article. M.B. Yurgelun has has Research funding from Janssen; and Consulting/scientific advisory board roles at Nouscom. Syngal has no disclosures related to this article. This study was supported by The Pancreatic Cancer Action Network Catalyst Award (N. Rodriguez) and the K12TR004381 award (N. Rodriguez) through Harvard Catalyst | The Harvard Clinical and Translational Science Center (National Center for Advancing Translational Sciences, National Institutes of Health). The content is solely the responsibility of the authors and does not necessarily represent the official views of Harvard Catalyst, Harvard University, and its affiliated academic health care centers, or the National Institutes of Health. This study was also supported by the Whittaker Family Fund, the Scragg Family Fund, and the Hooley Fund-Lynch Syndrome.

REFERENCES

1. Siegel RL, Miller KD, Wagle NS, et al. Cancer statistics, 2023. CA Cancer J Clin 2023;73(1):17–48.
2. Syngal S, Brand RE, Church JM, et al, American College of Gastroenterology. ACG clinical guideline: Genetic testing and management of hereditary gastrointestinal cancer syndromes. Am J Gastroenterol 2015;110(2):223–62, quiz 63.
3. Hassanin E, Spier I, Bobbili DR, et al. Clinically relevant combined effect of polygenic background, rare pathogenic germline variants, and family history on colorectal cancer incidence. BMC Med Genomics 2023;16(1):42.
4. Vilar E, Gruber SB. Microsatellite instability in colorectal cancer-the stable evidence. Nat Rev Clin Oncol 2010;7(3):153–62.
5. Win AK, Jenkins MA, Dowty JG, et al. Prevalence and penetrance of major genes and polygenes for colorectal cancer. Cancer Epidemiol Biomarkers Prev 2017;26(3):404–12.
6. Haraldsdottir S, Rafnar T, Frankel WL, et al. Comprehensive population-wide analysis of Lynch syndrome in Iceland reveals founder mutations in MSH6 and PMS2. Nat Commun 2017;8:14755.
7. Rosenblum RE, Ang C, Suckiel SA, et al. Lynch syndrome-associated variants and cancer rates in an ancestrally diverse biobank. JCO Precis Oncol 2020;4.
8. Grzymski JJ, Elhanan G, Morales Rosado JA, et al. Population genetic screening efficiently identifies carriers of autosomal dominant diseases. Nat Med 2020;26(8):1235–9.
9. Abu-Ghazaleh N, Kaushik V, Gorelik A, et al. Worldwide prevalence of Lynch syndrome in patients with colorectal cancer: systematic review and meta-analysis. Genet Med 2022;24(5):971–85.
10. Castellsagué E, Liu J, Volenik A, et al. Characterization of a novel founder MSH6 mutation causing Lynch syndrome in the French Canadian population. Clin Genet 2015;87(6):536–42.
11. Biller LH, Syngal S, Yurgelun MB. Recent advances in lynch syndrome. Fam Cancer 2019;18(2):211–9.

12. Dominguez-Valentin M, Sampson JR, Seppälä TT, et al. Cancer risks by gene, age, and gender in 6350 carriers of pathogenic mismatch repair variants: findings from the prospective lynch syndrome database. Genet Med 2020;22(1): 15–25.

13. Biller LH, Horiguchi M, Uno H, et al. Familial burden and other clinical factors associated with various types of cancer in individuals with lynch syndrome. Gastroenterology 2021;161(1):143–50.e4.

14. Biller LH, Creedon SA, Klehm M, et al. Lynch syndrome-associated cancers beyond colorectal cancer. Gastrointest Endosc Clin N Am 2022;32(1):75–93.

15. Network NCC. NCCN clinical practice guidelines in oncology (nccn guidelines®): genetic/familial high-risk assessment: colorectal version. 2. 2023. Available at: https://www.nccn.org/professionals/physician_gls/pdf/genetics_colon.pdf.

16. Lindor NM, Petersen GM, Hadley DW, et al. Recommendations for the care of individuals with an inherited predisposition to Lynch syndrome: a systematic review. JAMA 2006;296(12):1507–17.

17. Ranganathan M, Sacca RE, Trottier M, et al. Prevalence and clinical implications of mismatch repair-proficient colorectal cancer in patients with lynch syndrome. JCO Precis Oncol 2023;7:e2200675.

18. Ahadova A, Gallon R, Gebert J, et al. Three molecular pathways model colorectal carcinogenesis in Lynch syndrome. Int J Cancer 2018;143(1):139–50.

19. Valle L. Lynch syndrome: a single hereditary cancer syndrome or multiple syndromes defined by different mismatch repair genes? Gastroenterology 2023; 165(1):20–3.

20. Dabir PD, Bruggeling CE, van der Post RS, et al. Microsatellite instability screening in colorectal adenomas to detect Lynch syndrome patients? A systematic review and meta-analysis. Eur J Hum Genet 2020;28(3):277–86.

21. Lee BCH, Robinson PS, Coorens THH, et al. Mutational landscape of normal epithelial cells in lynch syndrome patients. Nat Commun 2022;13(1):2710.

22. Kloor M, Huth C, Voigt AY, et al. Prevalence of mismatch repair-deficient crypt foci in Lynch syndrome: a pathological study. Lancet Oncol 2012;13(6):598–606.

23. Pai RK, Dudley B, Karloski E, et al. DNA mismatch repair protein deficient non-neoplastic colonic crypts: a novel indicator of Lynch syndrome. Mod Pathol 2018;31(10):1608–18.

24. Ditonno I, Novielli D, Celiberto F, et al. Molecular pathways of carcinogenesis in familial adenomatous polyposis. Int J Mol Sci 2023;24(6).

25. Ahadova A, Stenzinger A, Seppälä T, et al, Lynpath Investigators. Two-in-One Hit" model of shortcut carcinogenesis in MLH1 lynch syndrome carriers. Gastroenterology 2023;165(1):267–70.e4.

26. Engel C, Ahadova A, Seppälä TT, et al, German HNPCC Consortium, the Dutch Lynch Syndrome Collaborative Group, Finnish Lynch Syndrome Registry. Associations of pathogenic variants in MLH1, MSH2, and MSH6 with risk of colorectal adenomas and tumors and with somatic mutations in patients with lynch syndrome. Gastroenterology 2020;158(5):1326–33.

27. Edelstein DL, Axilbund J, Baxter M, et al. Rapid development of colorectal neoplasia in patients with Lynch syndrome. Clin Gastroenterol Hepatol 2011; 9(4):340–3.

28. Monahan KJ, Swinyard O, Latchford A. Biology of precancers and opportunities for cancer interception: lesson from colorectal cancer susceptibility syndromes. Cancer Prev Res 2023;16(8):421–7.

29. Sánchez A, Roos VH, Navarro M, et al. Quality of colonoscopy is associated with adenoma detection and postcolonoscopy colorectal cancer prevention in lynch syndrome. Clin Gastroenterol Hepatol 2022;20(3):611–21.e9.
30. Vedantam S, Katona BW, Sussman DA, et al. Outcomes of upper endoscopy screening in Lynch syndrome: a meta-analysis. Gastrointest Endosc 2023; 97(1):2–10.e1.
31. Kumar S, Dudzik CM, Reed M, et al. Upper endoscopic surveillance in lynch syndrome detects gastric and duodenal adenocarcinomas. Cancer Prev Res 2020;13(12):1047–54.
32. Ceravolo AH, Yang JJ, Latham A, et al. Effectiveness of a surveillance program of upper endoscopy for upper gastrointestinal cancers in Lynch syndrome patients. Int J Colorectal Dis 2022;37(1):231–8.
33. Burn J, Sheth H, Elliott F, et al, CAPP2 Investigators. Cancer prevention with aspirin in hereditary colorectal cancer (Lynch syndrome), 10-year follow-up and registry-based 20-year data in the CAPP2 study: a double-blind, randomised, placebo-controlled trial. Lancet 2020;395(10240):1855–63.
34. Burn J, Gerdes AM, Macrae F, et al, CAPP2 Investigators. Long-term effect of aspirin on cancer risk in carriers of hereditary colorectal cancer: an analysis from the CAPP2 randomised controlled trial. Lancet 2011;378(9809):2081–7.
35. Mathers JC, Elliott F, Macrae F, et al, CAPP2 Investigators. Cancer Prevention with Resistant Starch in Lynch Syndrome Patients in the CAPP2-randomized placebo controlled trial: planned 10-year follow-up. Cancer Prev Res 2022;15(9): 623–34.
36. Willis JA, Reyes-Uribe L, Chang K, et al. Immune activation in mismatch repair-deficient carcinogenesis: more than just mutational rate. Clin Cancer Res 2020; 26(1):11–7.
37. Le DT, Kim TW, Van Cutsem E, et al. Phase II open-label study of pembrolizumab in treatment-refractory, microsatellite instability-high/mismatch repair-deficient metastatic colorectal cancer: KEYNOTE-164. J Clin Oncol 2020;38(1):11–9.
38. Le DT, Uram JN, Wang H, et al. PD-1 blockade in tumors with mismatch-repair deficiency. N Engl J Med 2015;372(26):2509–20.
39. Harrold EC, Foote MB, Rousseau B, et al. Neoplasia risk in patients with Lynch syndrome treated with immune checkpoint blockade. Nat Med 2023;29(10): 2458–63.
40. Sei S, Ahadova A, Keskin DB, et al. Lynch syndrome cancer vaccines: A roadmap for the development of precision immunoprevention strategies. Front Oncol 2023;13:1147590.
41. Hampel H, Kalady MF, Pearlman R, et al. Hereditary colorectal cancer. Hematol Oncol Clin N Am 2022;36(3):429–47.
42. Valle L, Monahan KJ. Genetic predisposition to gastrointestinal polyposis: syndromes, tumour features, genetic testing, and clinical management. Lancet Gastroenterol Hepatol 2024;9(1):68–82.
43. Sieber OM, Segditsas S, Knudsen AL, et al. Disease severity and genetic pathways in attenuated familial adenomatous polyposis vary greatly but depend on the site of the germline mutation. Gut 2006;55(10):1440–8.
44. Mankaney G, Leone P, Cruise M, et al. Gastric cancer in FAP: a concerning rise in incidence. Fam Cancer 2017;16(3):371–6.
45. Park SY, Ryu JK, Park JH, et al. Prevalence of gastric and duodenal polyps and risk factors for duodenal neoplasm in korean patients with familial adenomatous polyposis. Gut Liver 2011;5(1):46–51.

46. Jagelman DG, DeCosse JJ, Bussey HJ. Upper gastrointestinal cancer in familial adenomatous polyposis. Lancet 1988;1(8595):1149–51.

47. Wood LD, Salaria SN, Cruise MW, et al. Upper GI tract lesions in familial adenomatous polyposis (FAP): enrichment of pyloric gland adenomas and other gastric and duodenal neoplasms. Am J Surg Pathol 2014;38(3):389–93.

48. Attard TM, Giglio P, Koppula S, et al. Brain tumors in individuals with familial adenomatous polyposis: a cancer registry experience and pooled case report analysis. Cancer 2007;109(4):761–6.

49. Chenbhanich J, Atsawarungruangkit A, Korpaisarn S, et al. Prevalence of thyroid diseases in familial adenomatous polyposis: a systematic review and meta-analysis. Fam Cancer 2019;18(1):53–62.

50. Kennedy RD, Potter DD, Moir CR, et al. The natural history of familial adenomatous polyposis syndrome: a 24 year review of a single center experience in screening, diagnosis, and outcomes. J Pediatr Surg 2014;49(1):82–6.

51. Lamlum H, Ilyas M, Rowan A, et al. The type of somatic mutation at APC in familial adenomatous polyposis is determined by the site of the germline mutation: a new facet to Knudson's 'two-hit' hypothesis. Nat Med 1999;5(9):1071–5.

52. Borras E, San Lucas FA, Chang K, et al. Genomic Landscape of Colorectal Mucosa and Adenomas. Cancer Prev Res 2016;9(6):417–27.

53. Bugter JM, Fenderico N, Maurice MM. Mutations and mechanisms of WNT pathway tumour suppressors in cancer. Nat Rev Cancer 2021;21(1):5–21.

54. Fearon ER, Vogelstein B. A genetic model for colorectal tumorigenesis. Cell 1990;61(5):759–67.

55. Vogelstein B, Fearon ER, Hamilton SR, et al. Genetic alterations during colorectal-tumor development. N Engl J Med 1988;319(9):525–32.

56. Li J, Wang R, Zhou X, et al. Genomic and transcriptomic profiling of carcinogenesis in patients with familial adenomatous polyposis. Gut 2020;69(7):1283–93.

57. Giardiello FM, Hamilton SR, Krush AJ, et al. Treatment of colonic and rectal adenomas with sulindac in familial adenomatous polyposis. N Engl J Med 1993; 328(18):1313–6.

58. Ishikawa H, Mutoh M, Sato Y, et al. Chemoprevention with low-dose aspirin, mesalazine, or both in patients with familial adenomatous polyposis without previous colectomy (J-FAPP Study IV): a multicentre, double-blind, randomised, two-by-two factorial design trial. Lancet Gastroenterol Hepatol 2021;6(6):474–81.

59. Samadder NJ, Kuwada SK, Boucher KM, et al. Association of sulindac and erlotinib vs placebo with colorectal neoplasia in familial adenomatous polyposis: secondary analysis of a randomized clinical trial. JAMA Oncol 2018;4(5):671–7.

60. Samadder NJ, Neklason DW, Boucher KM, et al. Effect of Sulindac and erlotinib vs placebo on duodenal neoplasia in familial adenomatous polyposis: a randomized clinical trial. JAMA 2016;315(12):1266–75.

61. Burke CA, Dekker E, Lynch P, et al. Eflornithine plus sulindac for prevention of progression in familial adenomatous polyposis. N Engl J Med 2020;383(11): 1028–39.

62. Lin JS, Perdue LA, Henrikson NB, et al. Screening for colorectal cancer: updated evidence report and systematic review for the US preventive services task force. JAMA 2021;325(19):1978–98.

63. Davidson KW, Barry MJ, Mangione CM, et al. Screening for colorectal cancer: US preventive services task force recommendation statement. JAMA 2021; 325(19):1965–77.

64. Shaukat A, Kahi CJ, Burke CA, et al. ACG clinical guidelines: colorectal cancer screening 2021. Am J Gastroenterol 2021;116(3):458–79.

65. Peterse EFP, Meester RGS, Siegel RL, et al. The impact of the rising colorectal cancer incidence in young adults on the optimal age to start screening: Micro-simulation analysis I to inform the American Cancer Society colorectal cancer screening guideline. Cancer 2018;124(14):2964–73.

66. Siegel RL, Fedewa SA, Anderson WF, et al. Colorectal cancer incidence patterns in the United States, 1974-2013. J Natl Cancer Inst 2017;109(8).

67. Gupta S, Lieberman D, Anderson JC, et al. Recommendations for follow-up after colonoscopy and polypectomy: a consensus update by the us multi-society task force on colorectal cancer. Gastroenterology 2020;158(4):1131–53.e5.

68. Siegel RL, Wagle NS, Cercek A, et al. Colorectal cancer statistics, 2023. CA Cancer J Clin 2023;73(3):233–54.

69. Chung DC, Gray DM 2nd, Singh H, et al. A cell-free DNA blood-based test for colorectal cancer screening. N Engl J Med 2024;390(11):973–83.

70. Imperiale TF, Porter K, Zella J, et al, BLUE-C Study Investigators. Next-generation multitarget stool DNA test for colorectal cancer screening. N Engl J Med 2024;390(11):984–93.

71. He X, Wu K, Ogino S, et al. Association between risk factors for colorectal cancer and risk of serrated polyps and conventional adenomas. Gastroenterology 2018;155(2):355–73.e18.

72. Guirguis-Blake JM, Evans CV, Perdue LA, et al. Aspirin use to prevent cardiovascular disease and colorectal cancer: updated evidence report and systematic review for the US preventive services task force. JAMA 2022;327(16): 1585–97.

73. Issaka RB, Chan AT, Gupta S. AGA clinical practice update on risk stratification for colorectal cancer screening and post-polypectomy surveillance: expert review. Gastroenterology 2023;165(5):1280–91.

74. Gini A, Meester RGS, Keshavarz H, et al. Cost-effectiveness of colonoscopy-based colorectal cancer screening in childhood cancer survivors. J Natl Cancer Inst 2019;111(11):1161–9.

75. Hadjiliadis D, Khoruts A, Zauber AG, et al, Cystic Fibrosis Colorectal Cancer Screening Task Force. Cystic fibrosis colorectal cancer screening consensus recommendations. Gastroenterology 2018;154(3):736–45.e14.

76. Biller LH, Ukaegbu C, Dhingra TG, et al. A multi-institutional cohort of therapy-associated polyposis in childhood and young adulthood cancer survivors. Cancer Prev Res 2020;13(3):291–8.

77. Eaden JA, Mayberry JF, British Society for Gastroenterology, et al. Guidelines for screening and surveillance of asymptomatic colorectal cancer in patients with inflammatory bowel disease. Gut 2002;51(Suppl 5):V10–2.

78. Cottet V, Jooste V, Fournel I, et al. Long-term risk of colorectal cancer after adenoma removal: a population-based cohort study. Gut 2012;61(8):1180–6.

79. Erichsen R, Baron JA, Hamilton-Dutoit SJ, et al. Increased risk of colorectal cancer development among patients with serrated polyps. Gastroenterology 2016; 150(4):895–902.e5.

80. Uson PLS Jr, Borad MJ, Ahn D, et al. Germline cancer testing in unselected patients with gastric and esophageal cancers: a multi-center prospective study. Dig Dis Sci 2022;67(11):5107–15.

81. Ku GY, Kemel Y, Maron SB, et al. Prevalence of germline alterations on targeted tumor-normal sequencing of esophagogastric cancer. JAMA Netw Open 2021; 4(7):e2114753.

82. Yap TA, Ashok A, Stoll J, et al. Prevalence of germline findings among tumors from cancer types lacking hereditary testing guidelines. JAMA Netw Open 2022;5(5):e2213070.

83. Petrovchich I, Ford JM. Genetic predisposition to gastric cancer. Semin Oncol 2016;43(5):554–9.

84. Hansford S, Kaurah P, Li-Chang H, et al. Hereditary diffuse gastric cancer syndrome: CDH1 mutations and beyond. JAMA Oncol 2015;1(1):23–32.

85. Blair VR, McLeod M, Carneiro F, et al. Hereditary diffuse gastric cancer: updated clinical practice guidelines. Lancet Oncol 2020;21(8):e386–97.

86. Roberts ME, Ranola JMO, Marshall ML, et al. Comparison of CDH1 penetrance estimates in clinically ascertained families vs families ascertained for multiple gastric cancers. JAMA Oncol 2019;5(9):1325–31.

87. Huynh JM, Laukaitis CM. Panel testing reveals nonsense and missense CDH1 mutations in families without hereditary diffuse gastric cancer. Mol Genet Genomic Med 2016;4(2):232–6.

88. Lowstuter K, Espenschied CR, Sturgeon D, et al. Unexpected CDH1 mutations identified on multigene panels pose clinical management challenges. JCO Precis Oncol 2017;1:1–12.

89. Coudert M, Drouet Y, Delhomelle H, et al. First estimates of diffuse gastric cancer risks for carriers of CTNNA1 germline pathogenic variants. J Med Genet 2022;59(12):1189–95.

90. Benusiglio PR, Colas C, Guillerm E, et al. Clinical implications of CTNNA1 germline mutations in asymptomatic carriers. Gastric Cancer 2019;22(4):899–903.

91. Lobo S, Benusiglio PR, Coulet F, et al. Cancer predisposition and germline CTNNA1 variants. Eur J Med Genet 2021;64(10):104316.

92. Majewski IJ, Kluijt I, Cats A, et al. An α-E-catenin (CTNNA1) mutation in hereditary diffuse gastric cancer. J Pathol 2013;229(4):621–9.

93. Network NCC. NCCN clinical practice guidelines in oncology (NCCN guidelines®): gastric cancer. Version 2.2023. 2023. Available at: https://www.nccn.org/professionals/physician_gls/pdf/gastric.pdf.

94. Asif B, Sarvestani AL, Gamble LA, et al. Cancer surveillance as an alternative to prophylactic total gastrectomy in hereditary diffuse gastric cancer: a prospective cohort study. Lancet Oncol 2023;24(4):383–91.

95. Lee CYC, Olivier A, Honing J, et al. Endoscopic surveillance with systematic random biopsy for the early diagnosis of hereditary diffuse gastric cancer: a prospective 16-year longitudinal cohort study. Lancet Oncol 2023;24(1):107–16.

96. van der Post RS, Vogelaar IP, Carneiro F, et al. Hereditary diffuse gastric cancer: updated clinical guidelines with an emphasis on germline CDH1 mutation carriers. J Med Genet 2015;52(6):361–74.

97. Ellis A, Risk JM, Maruthappu T, et al. Tylosis with oesophageal cancer: Diagnosis, management and molecular mechanisms. Orphanet J Rare Dis 2015;10:126.

98. Blaydon DC, Etheridge SL, Risk JM, et al. RHBDF2 mutations are associated with tylosis, a familial esophageal cancer syndrome. Am J Hum Genet 2012;90(2):340–6.

99. Ellis A, Field JK, Field EA, et al. Tylosis associated with carcinoma of the oesophagus and oral leukoplakia in a large Liverpool family–a review of six generations. Eur J Cancer B Oral Oncol 1994;30b(2):102–12.

100. Sugrañes TA, Flanagan M, Thomas C, et al. Age of first cancer diagnosis and survival in Bloom syndrome. Genet Med 2022;24(7):1476–84.

101. Rosenberg PS, Socié G, Alter BP, et al. Risk of head and neck squamous cell cancer and death in patients with Fanconi anemia who did and did not receive transplants. Blood 2005;105(1):67–73.

102. Network NCC. NCCN clinical practice guidelines in oncology (NCCN Guidelines®): esophageal and esophagogastric junction cancers. Version 3.2023. 2023. Available at: https://www.nccn.org/professionals/physician_gls/pdf/esophageal.pdf.

103. Lee M, Eng G, Handte-Reinecker A, et al. Germline determinants of esophageal adenocarcinoma. Gastroenterology 2023;165(5):1276–9.e7.

104. Jencks DS, Adam JD, Borum ML, et al. Overview of current concepts in gastric intestinal metaplasia and gastric cancer. Gastroenterol Hepatol (N Y) 2018; 14(2):92–101.

105. Gupta S, Li D, El Serag HB, et al. AGA clinical practice guidelines on management of gastric intestinal metaplasia. Gastroenterology 2020;158(3):693–702.

106. Altayar O, Davitkov P, Shah SC, et al. AGA technical review on gastric intestinal metaplasia-epidemiology and risk factors. Gastroenterology 2020;158(3): 732–44.e16.

107. Gawron AJ, Shah SC, Altayar O, et al. AGA technical review on gastric intestinal metaplasia-natural history and clinical outcomes. Gastroenterology 2020; 158(3):705–31.e5.

108. Shin WS, Xie F, Chen B, et al. Updated epidemiology of gastric cancer in asia: decreased incidence but still a big challenge. Cancers (Basel) 2023;15(9).

109. Zhang X, Li M, Chen S, et al. Endoscopic screening in asian countries is associated with reduced gastric cancer mortality: a meta-analysis and systematic review. Gastroenterology 2018;155(2):347–54.e9.

110. Gupta S, Tao L, Murphy JD, et al. Race/ethnicity-socioeconomic status-and anatomic subsite-specific risks for gastric cancer. Gastroenterology 2019; 156(1):59–62.e4.

111. BARRETT NR. Chronic peptic ulcer of the oesophagus and 'oesophagitis'. Br J Surg 1950;38(150):175–82.

112. Shaheen NJ, Falk GW, Iyer PG, et al. Diagnosis and management of barrett's esophagus: an updated ACG guideline. Am J Gastroenterol 2022;117(4):559–87.

113. Winters C, Spurling TJ, Chobanian SJ, et al. Barrett's esophagus. A prevalent, occult complication of gastroesophageal reflux disease. Gastroenterology 1987;92(1):118–24.

114. Qumseya BJ, Bukannan A, Gendy S, et al. Systematic review and meta-analysis of prevalence and risk factors for Barrett's esophagus. Gastrointest Endosc 2019;90(5):707–17.e1.

115. Souza RF, Spechler SJ. Mechanisms and pathophysiology of Barrett oesophagus. Nat Rev Gastroenterol Hepatol 2022;19(9):605–20.

116. Hirota WK, Loughney TM, Lazas DJ, et al. Specialized intestinal metaplasia, dysplasia, and cancer of the esophagus and esophagogastric junction: prevalence and clinical data. Gastroenterology 1999;116(2):277–85.

117. Cameron AJ, Zinsmeister AR, Ballard DJ, et al. Prevalence of columnar-lined (Barrett's) esophagus. Comparison of population-based clinical and autopsy findings. Gastroenterology 1990;99(4):918–22.

118. Ormsby AH, Kilgore SP, Goldblum JR, et al. The location and frequency of intestinal metaplasia at the esophagogastric junction in 223 consecutive autopsies: implications for patient treatment and preventive strategies in Barrett's esophagus. Mod Pathol 2000;13(6):614–20.

119. Gerson LB, Shetler K, Triadafilopoulos G. Prevalence of Barrett's esophagus in asymptomatic individuals. Gastroenterology 2002;123(2):461–7.
120. Ward EM, Wolfsen HC, Achem SR, et al. Barrett's esophagus is common in older men and women undergoing screening colonoscopy regardless of reflux symptoms. Am J Gastroenterol 2006;101(1):12–7.
121. Cook MB, Coburn SB, Lam JR, et al. Cancer incidence and mortality risks in a large US Barrett's oesophagus cohort. Gut 2018;67(3):418–529.
122. Rastogi A, Puli S, El-Serag HB, et al. Incidence of esophageal adenocarcinoma in patients with Barrett's esophagus and high-grade dysplasia: a meta-analysis. Gastrointest Endosc 2008;67(3):394–8.
123. Wang A, Mattek NC, Holub JL, et al. Prevalence of complicated gastroesophageal reflux disease and Barrett's esophagus among racial groups in a multicenter consortium. Dig Dis Sci 2009;54(5):964–71.
124. Katz PO, Dunbar KB, Schnoll-Sussman FH, et al. ACG clinical guideline for the diagnosis and management of gastroesophageal reflux disease. Am J Gastroenterol 2022;117(1):27–56.
125. Spechler SJ, Sharma P, Souza RF, et al. American Gastroenterological Association medical position statement on the management of Barrett's esophagus. Gastroenterology 2011;140(3):1084–91.
126. Qumseya B, Sultan S, Bain P, et al, ASGE Standards of Practice Committee Chair. ASGE guideline on screening and surveillance of Barrett's esophagus. Gastrointest Endosc 2019;90(3):335–59.e2.
127. Sharma P, Shaheen NJ, Katzka D, et al. AGA clinical practice update on endoscopic treatment of barrett's esophagus with dysplasia and/or early cancer: expert review. Gastroenterology 2020;158(3):760–9.
128. Shah SL, Dunbar K. Revisiting proton pump inhibitors as chemoprophylaxis against the progression of barrett's esophagus. Curr Gastroenterol Rep 2023; 25(12):374–9.
129. Yurgelun MB, Chittenden AB, Morales-Oyarvide V, et al. Germline cancer susceptibility gene variants, somatic second hits, and survival outcomes in patients with resected pancreatic cancer. Genet Med 2019;21(1):213–23.
130. Hu C, Hart SN, Polley EC, et al. Association between inherited germline mutations in cancer predisposition genes and risk of pancreatic cancer. JAMA 2018;319(23):2401–9.
131. Shindo K, Yu J, Suenaga M, et al. Deleterious germline mutations in patients with apparently sporadic pancreatic adenocarcinoma. J Clin Oncol 2017;35(30): 3382–90.
132. Aslanian HR, Lee JH, Canto MI. AGA clinical practice update on pancreas cancer screening in high-risk individuals: expert review. Gastroenterology 2020; 159(1):358–62.
133. Network NCC. NCCN clinical practice guidelines in oncology (NCCN Guidelines®): genetic/familial high-risk assessment: breast, ovarian, and pancreatic. version 2.2024 — september 27, 2023. 2023. Available at: https://www.nccn.org/professionals/physician_gls/pdf/genetics_bop.pdf.
134. Wood LD, Yurgelun MB, Goggins MG. Genetics of familial and sporadic pancreatic cancer. Gastroenterology 2019;156(7):2041–55.
135. Seppälä TT, Burkhart RA, Katona BW. Hereditary colorectal, gastric, and pancreatic cancer: comprehensive review. BJS Open 2023;7(3):zrad023.
136. Semaan A, Bernard V, Wong J, et al. Integrated molecular characterization of intraductal papillary mucinous neoplasms: An NCI cancer moonshot precancer atlas pilot project. Cancer Res Commun 2023;3(10):2062–73.

137. Dbouk M, Katona BW, Brand RE, et al. The multicenter cancer of pancreas screening study: impact on stage and survival. J Clin Oncol 2022;40(28):3257–66.
138. Lennon AM, Wolfgang CL, Canto MI, et al. The early detection of pancreatic cancer: what will it take to diagnose and treat curable pancreatic neoplasia? Cancer Res 2014;74(13):3381–9.
139. Canto MI, Kerdsirichairat T, Yeo CJ, et al. Surgical outcomes after pancreatic resection of screening-detected lesions in individuals at high risk for developing pancreatic cancer. J Gastrointest Surg 2020;24(5):1101–10.
140. Yurgelun MB. Building on more than 20 years of progress in pancreatic cancer surveillance for high-risk individuals. J Clin Oncol 2022;40(28):3230–4.
141. Lucas AL, Fu Y, Labiner AJ, et al. Frequent abnormal pancreas imaging in patients with pathogenic ATM, BRCA1, BRCA2, and PALB2 breast cancer susceptibility variants. Clin Gastroenterol Hepatol 2023;21(10):2686–8.e2.
142. Shah I, Silva-Santisteban A, Germansky KA, et al. Pancreatic cancer screening for at-risk individuals (pancreas scan study): yield, harms, and outcomes from a prospective multicenter study. Am J Gastroenterol 2023;118(9):1664–70.
143. Calderwood AH, Sawhney MS, Thosani NC, et al. American Society for Gastrointestinal Endoscopy guideline on screening for pancreatic cancer in individuals with genetic susceptibility: methodology and review of evidence. Gastrointest Endosc 2022;95(5):827–54.e3.
144. Paiella S, Salvia R, De Pastena M, et al. Screening/surveillance programs for pancreatic cancer in familial high-risk individuals: A systematic review and proportion meta-analysis of screening results. Pancreatology 2018;18(4):420–8.
145. Haldar SD, Vilar E, Maitra A, et al. Worth a pound of cure? emerging strategies and challenges in cancer immunoprevention. Cancer Prev Res 2023;16(9): 483–95.
146. Fonseca AL, Kirkwood K, Kim MP, et al. Intraductal papillary mucinous neoplasms of the pancreas: current understanding and future directions for stratification of malignancy risk. Pancreas 2018;47(3):272–9.
147. Lee KS, Sekhar A, Rofsky NM, et al. Prevalence of incidental pancreatic cysts in the adult population on MR imaging. Am J Gastroenterol 2010;105(9):2079–84.
148. Laffan TA, Horton KM, Klein AP, et al. Prevalence of unsuspected pancreatic cysts on MDCT. AJR Am J Roentgenol 2008;191(3):802–7.
149. Crippa S, Fernández-Del Castillo C, Salvia R, et al. Mucin-producing neoplasms of the pancreas: an analysis of distinguishing clinical and epidemiologic characteristics. Clin Gastroenterol Hepatol 2010;8(2):213–9.
150. Tanaka M, Fernández-Del Castillo C, Kamisawa T, et al. Revisions of international consensus Fukuoka guidelines for the management of IPMN of the pancreas. Pancreatology 2017;17(5):738–53.
151. Elta GH, Enestvedt BK, Sauer BG, et al. ACG clinical guideline: diagnosis and management of pancreatic cysts. Am J Gastroenterol 2018;113(4):464–79.
152. Vege SS, Ziring B, Jain R, et al. American gastroenterological association institute guideline on the diagnosis and management of asymptomatic neoplastic pancreatic cysts. Gastroenterology 2015;148(4):819–22, quize12-3.
153. ESGoCTot Pancreas. European evidence-based guidelines on pancreatic cystic neoplasms. Gut 2018;67(5):789–804.
154. Ohtsuka T, Fernandez-Del Castillo C, Furukawa T, et al. International evidence-based Kyoto guidelines for the management of intraductal papillary mucinous neoplasm of the pancreas. Pancreatology 2023;24(2):255–70.

Cancer Precursor Syndromes and Their Detection in the Head and Neck

Alessandro Villa, DDS, PhD, MPH[a,b], William N. William Jr, MD[c], Glenn J. Hanna, MD[d,*]

KEYWORDS

- Oral cavity cancer • Oral potentially malignant disorders • Dyskeratosis congenita
- Fanconi anemia • Risk factors • Genetics

KEY POINTS

- Oral cavity cancer: Tobacco use, alcohol consumption are the main risk factors for oral cancer, along with genetic factors and immunosuppression.
- Hereditary conditions: Inherited disorders, such as dyskeratosis congenita and Fanconi anemia, increase the risk of oral cancer, necessitating specialized care and surveillance.
- Oral potentially malignant disorders (OPMDs): Conditions like leukoplakia serve as precursors to oral cancer, with genetic, immunologic, and molecular factors influencing progression, requiring personalized management strategies.
- Molecular and immunologic features: Genetic mutations, allelic imbalances, and immune modulation play critical roles in OPMD development, offering potential targets for therapeutic interventions and precision medicine.
- Therapeutic strategies and cancer prevention: Controversial management of oral precancers involves surgical resection, chemoprevention, and immune modulation; challenges persist in developing effective, evidence-based approaches for chemoprevention.

INTRODUCTION

Head and neck cancers represent a group of histopathologic malignancies arising in the oral cavity, pharynx, larynx, nasal cavity, paranasal sinuses, thyroid, and salivary glands which each have distinct epidemiologic associations and clinical behavior.

[a] Oral Medicine, Oral Oncology and Dentistry, Miami Cancer Institute, Baptist Health South Florida, 8900 N. Kendall Drive. Miami, FL 33176, USA; [b] Herbert Wertheim College of Medicine, Florida International University, Miami, FL, USA; [c] Thoracic Oncology Program, Grupo Oncoclínicas Grupo Oncoclínicas, Av. Pres. Juscelino Kubitschek, 510, 2º andar, São Paulo, São Paulo 04543-906, Brazil; [d] Department of Medical Oncology, Center for Head & Neck Oncology, Dana-Farber Cancer Institute, Harvard Medical School, 450 Brookline Avenue, Dana Building, Room 2-140. Boston, MA 02215, USA
* Corresponding author.
E-mail address: glenn_hanna@dfci.harvard.edu

Hematol Oncol Clin N Am 38 (2024) 813–830
https://doi.org/10.1016/j.hoc.2024.04.001
0889-8588/24/© 2024 Elsevier Inc. All rights reserved.

Wide geographic variation exists in terms of the incidence of primary head and neck cancers, which largely reflects risk factor heterogeneity among subpopulations. Squamous cell carcinoma (SCC) represents the most common histologic subtype arising from several aerodigestive mucosal regions. Stratified squamous epithelium that lines the majority of the oral cavity and other mucosal sites can sometimes give rise to premalignant oral lesions, or precursors to oral cancer of the head and neck. Here, we review the epidemiology, risk factors, and genetic syndromes that predispose to oral cancer, explore the molecular and immunologic underpinnings driving malignant oral transformation, and discuss the therapeutic strategies for oral cancer prevention and early interception.

EPIDEMIOLOGY AND RISK FACTORS

Oral cavity cancer (OCC) is a collection of malignancies arising from the mucosal subsites of the mouth often manifesting from squamous epithelial tissue, such as that more than 90% of cases are oral cavity SCCs.[1] There are nearly 400,000 cases of OCC diagnosed annually across the globe and more than 170,000 people die from these cancers each year.[2] Contributing factors for the development of OCC are described in the following sections, with consumption of tobacco products being the most important preventable risk factor.

Tobacco

Tobacco contains the addictive substance nicotine and carcinogens, such that smokers have more than 8 fold risk of developing oral cancer.[3] There is a firm association between smoking tobacco and oral cancer, with the most important carcinogens being aromatic hydrocarbon benzo-pyrene and the tobacco-specific nitrosamines namely 4-(nitrosomethylamino)-1-(3-pyridyl)-1-butanone (NNK) and N'-nitrosonornicotine (NNN). The metabolites of NNK and NNN bind DNA within oral mucosal keratinocytes leading to mutagenesis.[4] Additionally, xenobiotic metabolizing enzymes found in the liver and aerodigestive mucosa are key in activating and degrading tobacco carcinogens.[5] These enzymes are polymorphic and determine individual risk and oral cancer susceptibility.[6] Beyond smoking tobacco, smokeless tobacco can be placed into contact with the oral mucosa where nicotine is absorbed and chronic mucosal injury and fibrosis occurs.[7] Chewing betel quid (or pan), which contains betel leaf, areca nut, slaked lime (releasing alkaloid from the areca nut producing a euphoric feeling), tobacco, and sometimes spices is a common practice across South and Southeast Asia, particularly in India. Some betel quid ingredients are toxic to cells and trigger cellular proliferation or DNA damage.[8]

Alcohol

Alcohol is implicated in oral carcinogenesis but as an independent factor its role is unclear while it is clearly synergistic (35 fold risk) with tobacco use in causing oral cancer.[9] Alcohol has been shown to increase the permeability of oral mucosa by epithelial atrophy, which leads to carcinogenic exposure.[10] The major metabolite in alcohol is acetaldehyde, which is oxidized and interferes with DNA synthesis and repair. Further, activity of the enzyme that metabolizes alcohol itself, alcohol dehydrogenase, can be impacted by the oral microbiota, and individual genetic polymorphisms have been identified in this enzyme and other metabolizing enzymes.[11,12] Systemically, alcohol triggers hepatic or liver damage, which can lead to cirrhotic changes that can block carcinogen detoxification. Chronic nutritional issues related to alcohol consumption can lead to nutrient deficiencies that also pose cancer risk.

Diet and Nutrition

Several dietary nutrients have specific mechanisms of action that variably impact the risk of oral cancer. Foods such as fruits, vegetables, curcumin, and green tea can reduce the risk of oral cancer, while a proinflammatory diet rich in red meat and fried foods can enhance risk.[13] Proinflammatory foods trigger the production of cytokines such as interleukin-6, C-reactive protein, and homocysteine. High dietary iron intake has also been linked with cancer risk given its importance in cell proliferation and metabolic processes, while nitrates and nitrites in natural red meats are toxic and when cooked can release heterocyclic amines and hydrocarbons that are carcinogenic.[14,15] On the contrary, evidence associating high consumption of fruits and vegetables with a lower risk of cancer appears dose-dependent. Antioxidants decrease reactive oxygen species while some compounds found in vegetables are thought to have antitumoral properties, such as glycates and indole-3-carbinol (inducing phase II enzymes), responsible for eliminating reactive oxygen species and mediating DNA repair.[16,17] Vegetables also contain high levels of micronutrients (beta-carotene, alpha-carotene, lycopene, vitamins A, C, and E) that alone or in combination can have anticancerous properties.[18]

Viral Infections

It is well established that oropharyngeal epithelial infection of high-risk subtypes of human papillomavirus (HPV), namely 16 and 18, leads to late viral oncoprotein (E6 and E7) expression.[19] These viral proteins inactivate tumor suppressors that can lead to oropharyngeal cancer arising in the tonsil or base of tongue. Oral HPV infection rates are estimated to be around 2% to 8% with HPV16 being most common and more often identified in men.[20,21] High-risk HPV infection may be present in 10% to 25% of oral cavity squamous cell cancers, but studies analyzing viral oncoprotein expression have shown low rates (<10%) among oral cavity tumors.[22,23] Epstein-Barr virus (EBV) can cause lymphoproliferative disease in the setting of immunosuppression, but a causal relationship between EBV and oral cancer is not established. Similarly, serum titers of herpes simplex virus have been shown to be higher among patients with oral cancer, but the role of the virus in oral carcinogenesis is not clear but may relate to chronic immunosuppression leading to an imbalance of immunity leading to oncogene overexpression.[24]

Immunosuppression

Immune suppression does appear to be a risk factor for the development of oral cancers. Though somewhat controversial, even chronic ulceration or traumatic exposure from poor oral hygiene or dental status has been suggested as a risk factor. The presence of competing risk (tobacco and alcohol use) complicates interpretation of existing data.[25]

Personal History of Oral Cancer

Head and neck cancer survivors have an increased risk of developing second primary oral cavity tumors as compared to the overall population,[26,27] largely attributed to the field cancerization concept, which states that adjacent tissue to tumor contains certain preneoplastic molecular alterations from prior carcinogenic exposure.[28] Further, prior definitive radiotherapy to the head and neck also poses risk of developing a second primary head and neck malignancy, typically decades after the index cancer event.[29]

HEREDITARY CONDITIONS
Dyskeratosis Congenita

Introduction and pathogenesis

Dyskeratosis congenita (DKC) is an inherited multisystem disease characterized by bone marrow failure due to mutations in the telomere maintenance pathway, a predisposition to cancer, pulmonary fibrosis, and nonhematologic abnormalities.[30]

The prevalence of DKC in the general population is unknown, but it is estimated to be around 1 in 1 million people and is more frequently diagnosed in children with a higher incidence in male individuals.[31] Roughly 2% to 5% of individuals with bone marrow failure are diagnosed with DKC.

Recent developments have uncovered pathogenic germline genetic variants in a minimum of 15 telomere biology genes linked to DKC with a wide spectrum of diseases associated with DKC called telomere biology disorders.[32,33] Certain variants of DKC may present with complex multisystem illnesses (such as Hoyeraal–Hreidarsson syndrome, Revesz syndrome, or Coats plus) during early childhood, while others may develop with fewer medical issues later in life.[34,35]

Various inheritance patterns have been identified in telomere biology disorders, depending on the specific gene involved. Mutations in genes such as ACD, PARN, RTEL1, TERC, TERT, TINF2, and NAF1 have been associated with autosomal dominant inheritance of the disease.[36,37] Mutations in ACD, CTC1, NHP2, NOP10, PARN, RTEL1, STN1, TERT, and WRAP53 have been linked to autosomal recessive transmission of the disease.[38–40] And the sole reported X-linked DKC syndrome involves mutations in the DKC1 gene.[41,42] DKC1 encodes the dyskerin protein, playing a pivotal role in stabilizing telomerase, an enzyme critical for maintaining telomere length.[43] In the absence of proteins like dyskerin, telomeres gradually shorten, leading cells to undergo apoptosis or senescence and triggering carcinogenesis, particularly in rapidly dividing cells.[30,44] The more clinically severe variants of DKC tend to exhibit the most significant reduction in telomere length.

Clinical characteristics and diagnosis

The classic form of DKC is characterized by a triad of lacy reticular cutaneous hyperpigmentation on the upper chest and neck, nail dystrophy, and oral leukoplakia. These findings tend to develop in childhood although they are not present in all patients affected by DKC. Classic DKC may be diagnosed in patients exhibiting either all 3 mucocutaneous features or any single feature from the triad, coupled with bone marrow failure and 2 other somatic features of DKC. In addition, patients with DKC are at risk of developing a variety of cancers including head and neck cancers (40%), esophageal and stomach cancer (17%), anorectal carcinoma and cutaneous cancers (12% each), acute leukemia (8%), and liver cancer (5%).[45,46] The emergence of bone marrow failure, myelodysplastic syndrome, or pulmonary fibrosis aligns with a confirmed pathogenic germline variant in a gene linked to telomere biology disorders.[47]

Diagnostic testing for DKC includes assessing telomere length and conducting genetic tests for specific mutations. The testing approach depends on the patient's presentation. For individuals with a de novo presentation or a family history suggestive of a telomere disorder, a flow-FISH is recommended to measure telomere length on peripheral blood lymphocytes using peptide nucleic acid probes.[48] An average telomere length below the first percentile for age indicates abnormally short telomeres, consistent with DKC or a related telomere biology disorders. Even in cases with a known familial mutation, telomere length analysis is recommended to assess the extent of DKC-related complications in family members. Patients suspected of having DKC based on clinical criteria and telomere length analysis should undergo genetic testing to identify causative mutations. This is crucial for establishing a genetic diagnosis, testing first-degree relatives for carrier or disease status, and determining their eligibility as stem cell donors. It is important to note that identifying a pathogenic DKC mutation (such as DKC1, TERC, TERT, NOP10, NHP2, TINF2, TCAB1 [WRAP53], CTC1, RTEL1, ACD [TPP1], PARN, POT1, STN1, NAF1, ZCCHC8, MDM4, RPA1, and DCLRE1B) is considered diagnostic, but negative genetic test results do not rule out the possibility of DKC, as some patients may have unknown variants.

Management
Patients diagnosed with DKC and related telomere biology disorders require a specialized and multidisciplinary approach. Patients with a new-onset bone marrow failure should be tested for Fanconi anemia (FA) through chromosome breakage analysis. If this test yields normal results, it is advisable to proceed with clinical telomere length testing. Supportive care through transfusions might become necessary for patients with severe anemia or thrombocytopenia.[49]

Allogeneic HSCT is currently the only curative treatment option for patients with hematopoietic and/or immunologic abnormalities, although it is associated with complications.[50] Given the increased DKC cancer risk, patients should avoid smoking, excessive sun exposure, and limit alcohol intake, especially post-HSCT. Genetic counseling during testing is recommended to guide decisions and prepare individuals for potential outcomes.

While the survival of patients with DKC has improved over time, it still remains low. Mortality in DKC predominantly stems from bone marrow failure and its related consequences, underlying once again the need for ongoing surveillance and prompt testing of family members to ascertain the potential for interventions or eligibility as donors.[51,52]

Fanconi Anemia

Introduction and pathogenesis
FA is a rare hereditary genetic condition affecting all 3 blood cell lines characterized by pancytopenia, an increased susceptibility to malignancies, and congenital malformations or unique physical abnormalities.[53] The prevalence rates range from 1 in 100,000 to 250,000 births with higher rates among African population of South Africa, sub-Saharan Blacks, Spanish Gitanos, and Ashkenazi Jews in the United States (birthrate 1: 30,000).[54–57]

FA is the most frequent cause of bone marrow failure among inherited conditions and is characterized by the disruption of DNA repair mechanisms, culminating in cell death, genomic instability, and aberrations in the cell cycle. Specifically, FA is characterized by an absence of DNA repair capability to eliminate a category of DNA lesions called interstrand cross-links (ICLs).[58] Due to the accumulation of ICLs in rapidly dividing cells, such as hematopoietic stem cells in the bone marrow, individuals with FA experience bone marrow failure and an increased risk of developing cancer. The pathogenesis of FA involves mutations in over 22 distinct genes. Predominantly, mutations in FANCC, FANCA, and FANCG account for 80% to 90% of FA cases, while FANCD1 gene mutations, though less frequent, exhibit unique attributes and an increased susceptibility to malignancies. Over 200 distinct pathogenic alleles of FANCA have been identified, contributing to the unique genetic profile within individual pedigrees.[59] In the FANCA group, patients with 2 mutations leading to null alleles, in contrast to those with at least one hypomorphic mutation, are at higher risk of developing myelodysplastic syndrome (MDS) and acute myeloid leukemia (AML), with a shorter survival after diagnosis and exhibit an earlier onset of hematologic abnormalities.[60] When comparing mutations in FANCA or FANCC to mutations in FANCG, similar frequencies of nonhematologic anomalies were observed. However, mutations in FANCG are linked to more pronounced cytopenias and elevated rates of hematologic malignancies compared to mutations in FANCA or FANCC.[60]

Clinical characteristics and diagnosis

Patients with FA are predisposed to malignancy, developmental anomalies, and cytopenia. Malformations have been described in 60% to 70% of patients. Bone marrow failure occurs in the majority of patients with FA with different time to onset. Patients are also at risk of MDS or AML, with a 6000 fold increase compared to the general population.[61] Additionally, patients with FA are susceptible to acute lymphoblastic leukemia and Burkitt lymphoma, alongside solid tumors including SCC of the head and neck (because of the heightened replicative capacity in these tissues, driving the progression of cancer), nongenital cancers, and basal cell carcinoma, with the risk increasing with age. In a study conducted by a 2018 analysis of The National Cancer Institute Inherited Bone Marrow Failure Syndromes cohort showed that solid tumors were diagnosed in 20% of young patients with FA with the most common being oral SCC, skin SCC, cutaneous basal cell carcinoma, and anogenital cancers.[62] A recent retrospective study of 105 patients with FA showed that 8.6% patients presented with oral leukoplakia or erythroplakia and 3.8% underwent malignant transformation.[63]

The clinical spectrum further extends to encompass various endocrine disorders, including diabetes, adrenal, thyroid, and gonadal dysfunction. Patients with FA often presents with congenital abnormalities known as VACTERL-H association and PHENOS.[62,64] VACTERL-H encompasses a spectrum of anomalies, including vertebral irregularities, anal atresia, cardiac defects, tracheoesophageal fistula, esophageal atresia, renal and radial abnormalities, limb anomalies, and hydrocephalus. On the other hand, PHENOS is characterized by skin pigmentations, a reduced head size, small eyes, nervous system anomalies, otology-related diseases, and short stature. Notably, these congenital anomalies do not exhibit a strong association with the development of cancer.[62,64]

In addition to a thorough history and physical examination, patients with a suspicious diagnosis of FA should undergo screening tests for defective DNA repair, and genetic testing aimed at identifying the specific genetic disorder. Once an FA diagnosis is made, all first-degree siblings should be tested, as the phenotype is variable within families, and it is common to see more than one child with FA in a family.

Screening tests for FA exhibit high sensitivity, although they lack specificity. A positive test result may also be observed in other inherited disorders characterized by chromosomal instability.[65] For definitive confirmation of the diagnosis, the use of next-generation sequencing is recommended especially for all patients who yield a positive result in the chromosomal breakage test.

HSCT remains the primary curative treatment of FA-associated bone marrow failure, MDS, and leukemia. For those awaiting or ineligible for HSCT, alternative treatments include anabolic steroids such as danazol, oxandrolone, and oxymetholone.[66] However, these options do not offer a definitive cure for bone marrow failure. While these treatments provide temporary improvement of blood counts, they necessitate repeated administration. Caution is advised against prolonged use of steroid treatments to mitigate the potential risks of side effects and clonal evolution.[67] Finally, due to the high risk of solid tumors, routine surveillance (including thorough oral examinations) and preventive measures are recommended.

ORAL POTENTIALLY MALIGNANT DISORDERS
Introduction and Pathogenesis

A proportion of oral cancers arise by precursor lesions called oral potentially malignant disorders (OPMDs) in a multistep process in which normal cells are transformed into preneoplastic cells and then to cancer.[68,69] OPMDs are defined by the World Health Organization (WHO) as oral conditions "that carry a risk of cancer development in the oral cavity, whether in a clinically definable precursor lesion or in clinically normal mucosa" and precede a proportion of oral SCC.[70,71] The most common prevalent OPMDs include oral submucous fibrosis, leukoplakia, lichen planus, and erythroplakia.[72,73] Oral submucous fibrosis is an insidious oral precancer commonly seen in Southeast Asian countries due to areca nut chewing with malignant transformation rates ranging from 1.9% to 9%.[74] Oral lichen planus is an immune-mediated condition with an overall transformation rate of 1.4%,[75] and erythroplakia is an erythematous plaque of the oral cavity characterized by a malignant transformation rate of approximately 20%.[76] For the purpose of this review, we focused on leukoplakia as it stands out as one of the most frequently observed and extensively researched OPMD.

Leukoplakia has been defined by the WHO as "a white plaque of questionable risk having excluded (other) known diseases or disorders that carry no increased risk for cancer."[77] The estimated pooled prevalence of oral leukoplakia in the general population ranges from 1.5% (1.4%–1.6%, 95% confidence interval [CI]) to 2.6% (1.7%–2.7%, 95% CI).[78] Risk factors for oral leukoplakia are similar to those observed in oral cancer and include tobacco smoking, heavy alcohol consumption, areca nut chewing, immunosuppression, personal or family history of cancer, oral chronic graft versus host disease, ultraviolet light exposure and selected syndromes, including DKC and FA.[79,80]

Clinical Characteristics and Diagnosis

Two different subtypes of oral leukoplakia exist: homogenous leukoplakia (also called localized leukoplakia), and nonhomogenous leukoplakia.[81] The homogenous type is usually characterized by well-defined margins and fissured lesions while the nonhomogenous leukoplakia shows verrucous/nodular lesions or erythro-leukoplakia (mixed red and white changes). Another subset of the nonhomogeneous leukoplakias is called proliferative verrucous leukoplakia (PVL), which is characterized by multifocal lesions at different sites, or a large leukoplakia.[82–84] These conditions not only show different clinical features but also are characterized by a different genetic profile and malignant transformation rates.[85–87] The malignant transformation of homogenous leukoplakia ranges from 7.7% to 22.0% while that for PVL is 70% to 100%.[70,88,89] As for other cancers, oral cancer is thought to progress through a series of well-defined histopathological stages (from hyperkeratosis nonreactive to mild, moderate, or severe epithelial dysplasia).[79,90,91] The incisional biopsy remains the gold standard for the diagnosis of leukoplakia.[81] A 2022 review study summarizing the literature on the malignant progression of oral leukoplakia showed that when the histopathological diagnosis was considered, patients with hyperkeratosis nonreactive had a malignant transformation of 4.9%, and those with epithelial dysplasia had a 15.3% rate.[92]

Management

Oral leukoplakia, especially the proliferative type (PVL), remains a challenging condition to treat.

Surgical excision is associated with recurrence rates ranging approximately from 10% to 35%.[93–95] Other modalities of treatment that have been reported include laser ablation, cryotherapy photodynamic therapy, and medical therapy (such as retinoids, bleomycin, adenovirus, and green tea/black raspberry gel).[96–100] However, none of these have been proven to be effective and showed high recurrence rates. A range of new approaches are currently being evaluated with some promising results.[101] These vary in formulation, route of administration, and biological target.

MOLECULAR AND IMMUNOLOGIC FEATURES

Oral precancers represent an excellent opportunity for the study of carcinogenesis, since these lesions are oftentimes clinically apparent (eg, leukoplakia and erythro-leukoplakia), and readily accessible for biopsies, thus allowing them to be monitored for malignant transformation in, what could be initially thought of as, a relatively straightforward way. Nonetheless, there have been significant challenges in developing a molecular and immunologic progression model of oral carcinogenesis. These difficulties arise because time to oral cancer development is long (hindering consistent clinical follow-up and serial sampling over time), signs and symptoms of malignant transformation are not uniform (and sometimes occult), tissue samples routinely obtained in clinical practice are minute (and frequently unsuitable for high throughput profiling), cancer risk is not absolute and extremely variable from individual to individual with precancer lesions (even when histologic features, such as dysplasia, have been identified),[102,103] and the oral carcinogenic process is multistep and multipath (therefore involving complex molecular interactions).

In 1996, Califano and colleagues published one of the first genetic models of oral precancers.[104] By evaluating allelic imbalances of 10 critical chromosomal loci enriched for tumor suppressor genes, they identified loss of 9p21, 3p21, and 17p13 as early events, and an increase in frequency and number of regions lost along the spectrum of hyperplastic lesions without dysplasia, lesions with dysplasia, carcinoma in situ, and invasive cancers. These data were confirmed by Mao and colleagues, showing an increased progression risk in individuals with oral leukoplakia harboring loss of heterozygosity (LOH) at 9p21 and/or 3p14.[105] The British Columbia Oral Cancer Prevention Program evaluated these genomic markers in individuals with precancers referred by a community network over more than a decade, in multiple retrospective and prospective cohorts. By and large, this series of studies corroborated and expanded on the previous findings, in individuals with precancers without[106,107] and with[108] a prior oral cancer history, and contributed to rendering allelic imbalances the most robust markers of oral precancer progression. These studies also formed the basis for the adoption of LOH as the molecular inclusion criterion in the first, randomized, molecularly-based precision medicine study of oral precancers—the Erlotinib Prevention of Oral Cancer (EPOC) trial.

In EPOC, individuals with oral precancers, without or with a prior history of oral cancer, were assessed for LOH at 3p14, 9p21, 17p, 8p, 11p, 4q, or 13q. Patients were considered high-risk if they either had a prior history of oral cancer and LOH at 3p14 and/or 9p21 or had LOH at 3p14 and/or 9p21 plus an additional chromosomal site in the absence of a prior cancer history. Only high-risk individuals were then randomized to receive erlotinib or placebo for 1 year. EPOC did not meet its primary endpoint of oral cancer-free survival. However, the study provided a unique opportunity to longitudinally and formally characterize precancer prognosis, and demonstrated LOH profiles to be associated with malignant transformation, with a 3 year oral cancer-free survival of 74% versus 87% in the high-risk versus low-risk groups, respectively (HR, 2.19; 95% CI, 1.25–3.83; $P = .01$).[109] A long-term update of the EPOC trial confirmed that, among all allelic imbalances, 9p loss was the strongest molecular risk marker for oral cancer, especially in the context of dysplastic precancer lesions.[110]

While somatic copy number alterations in oral precancers have been more extensively characterized over the last 3 decades, and continue to be improved upon as key markers of cancer risk,[111] profiling of somatic mutations lagged behind, even though it has become a cornerstone of modern precision oncology. It was not until 2018 that a large-scale comprehensive evaluation of the mutational landscape of oral precancers was reported, along with its prognostic significance.[112] Using prospectively collected samples from patients with a median of 7.3 years of follow-up, William and colleagues showed (1) an increase in precancer lesion mutational burden from samples without dysplasia, to samples with dysplasia, to samples showing the development of invasive oral cancers; (2) a positive association between allelic imbalances and mutational load; (3) a higher oral cancer risk in lesions with high mutational load; and (4) similar mutation patterns of oral precancers compared to cancers, albeit at lower frequencies—most common mutations found in precancers were in *TP53* (29%), followed by *CDKN2A*, *NOTCH1*, *PIK3CA*, *KMT2D*, and *CASP8*. Importantly, *TP53* mutations were associated with an increased oral cancer risk (HR, 1.73; 95% CI, 1.07–2.78; P = .0250), and together with dysplasia and allelic imbalances, significantly contributed to predicting 5 year oral cancer-free survival in a multivariable histopathologic-genomic model (5 year oral cancer-free survival of 47% in the high-risk group with all 3 alterations vs 81% in the low-risk, no dysplasia group). Wils and colleagues, using a separate cohort, also recently demonstrated mutations in *TP53*, *FAT1*, *NOTCH1*, *CDKN2A*, and *PIK3CA* to be among the top 5 present in oral precancers.[113]

Fueled by the important therapeutic role of PD-1 inhibition in advanced head and neck SCCs, there has been renewed interest in studying the immune profile of oral precancers. Early small-scale studies showed abundance of T cells in subepithelial layers of oral precancers, especially in the context of dysplasia,[114,115] and in some cases associated with a lower risk of malignant transformation,[116] suggesting existence of immune surveillance even at the preinvasive stage. These findings were expanded upon by several groups, including the evaluation of the PD-1/PD-L1 axis. Collectively, these data showed PD-L1 expression in oral precancers (at lower frequencies compared to invasive cancers),[85,117–119] generally associated with an increased risk of malignant transformation.[117–119] In one of the largest data sets reported to date, using multiplex immunofluorescence, evidence for an inflamed phenotype of oral precancers was observed (characterized by positive correlations between precancer T cell infiltration, macrophage infiltration, and PD-L1 expression in epithelial and immune cells).[119] The lowest oral cancer-free survival rates were seen with lesions exhibiting high PD-L1 expression and low CD8+ T-cell infiltration (a pattern termed intrinsic induction).[119] Transcriptomic-based immune cell type deconvolution studies also showed immune and inflamed phenotypes in a subset of oral precancers.[120] PVLs were found to distinctly harbor abundant CD8+ T cells and T regulatory cells, along with PD-L1 upregulation, which could contribute to their high risk of malignant transformation.[85] Taken together, these results corroborate the role of immune evasion in oral carcinogenesis and pave the way for the evaluation of immune modulatory strategies for cancer prevention.

The mechanisms triggering precancer immune evasion have not been completely elucidated. The interplay between genomic alterations, immune escape, and malignant transformation is likely complex, and possibly involves chromosome 9p, a hotbed for immune genes such as *CD274* encoding PD-L1, *PD-L2*, *JAK2*, and interferons. In HPV-negative invasive head and neck cancers, 9p loss was demonstrated to be associated with an immune-cold phenotype and resistance to PD-1 inhibitors.[110,121] Conversely, in precancers, 9p loss was found to be associated with an increased T cell infiltration but augmented the risk of malignant transformation. We have recently proposed a model, according to which an aneuploid switch occurs promoting an immune hot-to-cold, precancer-to-cancer transition, possibly mediated by an increase in the deletion size of parts of chromosome 9p, co-occurring mutations (such as in *TP53*), and/or epistatic interactions with other genes.[110] Further characterization of this model may help elucidate precancer immunogenomics, as well as support precision immune prevention interventions.

THERAPEUTIC STRATEGIES AND CANCER PREVENTION DRUG DEVELOPMENT

Management of oral precancers is controversial, given that no therapeutic intervention has been consistently shown to reduce the risk of oral cancer long term.[122,123] The presence of high-grade dysplasia has been used as the major criterion to recommend surgical resection of oral precancers, even though (retrospective) studies have shown conflicting results of the impact of surgical intervention on long-term outcomes.[122] One of the shortcomings of local therapy in this setting stems from the field cancerization effect,[124] which makes it practically impossible to treat the widespread, histopathologically and/or molecularly abnormal mucosa at risk, even when detectable lesions are completely excised. Delivery of topical or systemic agents (eg, chemoprevention) might be a way to overcome this limitation and has been the subject of clinical investigation over the last several decades. Unfortunately, none of the trials performed to date resulted in development of a standard-of-care pharmacologic approach for oral cancer prevention.

A complete description of pharmacologic strategies is beyond the scope of this text. Reviews on this topic have been recently published.[96,100] It is worth highlighting, however, that drug development in this context is not without its challenges. Many clinical trials have used clinical or histopathological response as their primary endpoint, yet there is limited (if any) data showing these to be appropriate surrogate markers for oral cancer-free survival. Studies that choose invasive cancer as an endpoint might require large sample sizes and long-term follow-up, as oral cancer development takes time, and is usually an infrequent event, even in the context of a precancer lesion. Until recently, the use of agents with activity in advanced invasive disease (and possibly with a higher likelihood of being effective in precancers) was not possible, given side effect profiles and inconvenient dosing schedules. Predictive biomarkers of efficacy from pharmacologic interventions are largely unidentified in advanced head and neck cancers, let alone in oral precancers. Lastly, there has been insufficient characterization of oral precancer biology (in vivo or in vitro) to guide clinical development.[125]

Our groups and others have attempted to address many of the aforementioned challenges in several fronts: in EPOC, one of the most recent randomized trials in oral-precancers, William and colleagues selected patients with high-risk precancer on the basis of molecular criteria, which allowed for a reduced sample size and duration of the trial, due to the high expected number of events. This also provided sufficient statistical power for oral cancer-free survival to be used as the study's primary endpoint.[109] Hanna and colleagues have also selected a high-risk population on the basis of a specific clinical scenario—PVL, which nearly universally leads to invasive cancer development. This was the first reported immunoprevention study in oral precancers, transitioning an approved PD-1 inhibitor (nivolumab) from the metastatic to the preinvasive setting.[101] Rationale for this approach included previous immune profiling studies in this setting[85] and evidence of activity of PD-1 blockade in preclinical experiments.[126] Pretreatment and posttreatment biopsies during the trial revealed novel insights into mechanisms of resistance to nivolumab-based immune prevention (including the role of 9p loss and upregulation of LAG3), illustrating the value of translational research embedded into signal-finding studies.[101] Wang and colleagues have refined animal models of oral precancers and cancers that strongly mimic tobacco-induced carcinogenic in humans,[127] while Errazquin and colleagues have developed a mouse for spontaneous oral precancer/cancer in FA.[128] There have been several efforts to optimize precancer in vitro tissue culture models as well.[129] It is our belief that application of these tools will accelerate the development of clinical chemo and/or immune prevention strategies in the near future.

CLINICS CARE POINTS

- Employ a multidisciplinary team for the management of oral precancers, recognizing the need for personalized treatment plans based on individual patient characteristics and risk profile.

- Despite challenges, ongoing research in evidence-based preventive approaches is needed for advancing oral precancer management and reducing the risk of malignant transformation.

- Patients with DKC and FA should be monitored carefully given the increased risk of secondary oral cancer.

DISCLOSURE

Dr G.J. Hanna receives research funding to his institution from Bristol-Myers Squibb, United States (BMS) and has served in an advisory role for BMS. The other authors have nothing to disclose.

REFERENCES

1. Sung H, Ferlay J, Siegel RL, et al. Global Cancer Statistics 2020: GLOBOCAN Estimates of Incidence and Mortality Worldwide for 36 Cancers in 185 Countries. CA Cancer J Clin 2021;71(3):209–49.
2. Rivera C. Essentials of oral cancer. Int J Clin Exp Pathol 2015;8(9):11884–94.
3. Lin WJ, Jiang RS, Wu SH, et al. Smoking, alcohol, and betel quid and oral cancer: a prospective cohort study. J Oncol 2011;2011:525976.
4. Gupta PC, Murti PR, Bhonsle RB, et al. Effect of cessation of tobacco use on the incidence of oral mucosal lesions in a 10-yr follow-up study of 12,212 users. Oral Dis 1995;1(1):54–8.
5. Warnakulasuriya KA, Johnson NW, Linklater KM, et al. Cancer of mouth, pharynx and nasopharynx in Asian and Chinese immigrants resident in Thames regions. Oral Oncol 1999;35(5):471–5.
6. Warnakulasuriya KA, Ralhan R. Clinical, pathological, cellular and molecular lesions caused by oral smokeless tobacco–a review. J Oral Pathol Med 2007; 36(2):63–77.
7. Axell T. Occurrence of leukoplakia and some other oral white lesions among 20,333 adult Swedish people. Community Dent Oral Epidemiol 1987;15(1): 46–51.
8. Hecht SS. Tobacco carcinogens, their biomarkers and tobacco-induced cancer. Nat Rev Cancer 2003;3(10):733–44.

9. Hashibe M, Brennan P, Benhamou S, et al. Alcohol drinking in never users of to-bacco, cigarette smoking in never drinkers, and the risk of head and neck can-cer: pooled analysis in the International Head and Neck Cancer Epidemiology Consortium. J Natl Cancer Inst 2007;99(10):777–89.

10. Jafarey NA, Mahmood Z, Zaidi SH. Habits and dietary pattern of cases of car-cinoma of the oral cavity and oropharynx. J Pak Med Assoc 1977;27(6):340–3.

11. Murti PR, Bhonsle RB, Pindborg JJ, et al. Malignant transformation rate in oral submucous fibrosis over a 17-year period. Community Dent Oral Epidemiol 1985;13(6):340–1.

12. Hashibe M, Mathew B, Kuruvilla B, et al. Chewing tobacco, alcohol, and the risk of erythroplakia. Cancer Epidemiol Biomarkers Prev 2000;9(7):639–45.

13. Rodriguez-Molinero J, Miguelanez-Medran BDC, Puente-Gutierrez C, et al. As-sociation between Oral Cancer and Diet: An Update. Nutrients 2021;13(4).

14. Hernandez JD, Castell A, Arroyo-Manzanares N, et al. Toward Nitrite-Free Curing: Evaluation of a New Approach to Distinguish Real Uncured Meat from Cured Meat Made with Nitrite. Foods 2021;10(2).

15. Mazul AL, Shivappa N, Hebert JR, et al. Proinflammatory diet is associated with increased risk of squamous cell head and neck cancer. Int J Cancer 2018; 143(7):1604–10.

16. Gonzales JF, Barnard ND, Jenkins DJ, et al. Applying the precautionary princi-ple to nutrition and cancer. J Am Coll Nutr 2014;33(3):239–46.

17. Glade MJ. Food, nutrition, and the prevention of cancer: a global perspective. American Institute for Cancer Research/World Cancer Research Fund, Amer-ican Institute for Cancer Research, 1997. Nutrition 1999;15(6):523–6.

18. Chainani-Wu N. Diet and oral, pharyngeal, and esophageal cancer. Nutr Cancer 2002;44(2):104–26.

19. Ke LD, Adler-Storthz K, Mitchell MF, et al. Expression of human papillomavirus E7 mRNA in human oral and cervical neoplasia and cell lines. Oral Oncol 1999;35(4):415–20.

20. Kreimer AR, Villa A, Nyitray AG, et al. The epidemiology of oral HPV infection among a multinational sample of healthy men. Cancer Epidemiol Biomarkers Prev 2011;20(1):172–82.

21. Ang KK, Harris J, Wheeler R, et al. Human papillomavirus and survival of pa-tients with oropharyngeal cancer. N Engl J Med 2010;363(1):24–35.

22. Lingen MW, Xiao W, Schmitt A, et al. Low etiologic fraction for high-risk human papillomavirus in oral cavity squamous cell carcinomas. Oral Oncol 2013; 49(1):1–8.

23. Gillison ML, Chaturvedi AK, Anderson WF, et al. Epidemiology of Human Papillomavirus-Positive Head and Neck Squamous Cell Carcinoma. J Clin Oncol 2015;33(29):3235–42.

24. Jain M. Assesment of Correlation of Herpes Simplex Virus-1 with Oral Cancer and Precancer- A Comparative Study. J Clin Diagn Res 2016;10(8):ZC14–7.

25. Perry BJ, Zammit AP, Lewandowski AW, et al. Sites of origin of oral cavity cancer in nonsmokers vs smokers: possible evidence of dental trauma carcinogenesis and its importance compared with human papillomavirus. JAMA Otolaryngol Head Neck Surg 2015;141(1):5–11.

26. Coca-Pelaz A, Rodrigo JP, Suarez C, et al. The risk of second primary tumors in head and neck cancer: A systematic review. Head Neck 2020;42(3):456–66.

27. Lu D, Zhou X, Sun H, et al. Risk of second primary cancer in patients with head and neck squamous cell carcinoma: a systemic review and meta-analysis. Clin Oral Investig 2023;27(9):4897–910.

28. Dakubo GD, Jakupciak JP, Birch-Machin MA, et al. Clinical implications and utility of field cancerization. Cancer Cell Int 2007;7:2.

29. Ng SP, Pollard C 3rd, Kamal M, et al. Risk of second primary malignancies in head and neck cancer patients treated with definitive radiotherapy. npj Precis Oncol 2019;3:22.

30. Kirwan M, Dokal I. Dyskeratosis congenita, stem cells and telomeres. Biochim Biophys Acta 2009;1792(4):371–9.

31. Kirwan M, Dokal I. Dyskeratosis congenita: a genetic disorder of many faces. Clin Genet 2008;73(2):103–12.

32. Niewisch MR, Savage SA. An update on the biology and management of dyskeratosis congenita and related telomere biology disorders. Expert Rev Hematol 2019;12(12):1037–52.

33. Niewisch MR, Giri N, McReynolds LJ, et al. Disease progression and clinical outcomes in telomere biology disorders. Blood 2022;139(12):1807–19.

34. Savage SA. Dyskeratosis congenita and telomere biology disorders. Hematology Am Soc Hematol Educ Program 2022;2022(1):637–48.

35. Deng Z, Glousker G, Molczan A, et al. Inherited mutations in the helicase RTEL1 cause telomere dysfunction and Hoyeraal-Hreidarsson syndrome. Proc Natl Acad Sci U S A. 2013;110(36):E3408–16.

36. Armanios M, Chen JL, Chang YP, et al. Haploinsufficiency of telomerase reverse transcriptase leads to anticipation in autosomal dominant dyskeratosis congenita. Proc Natl Acad Sci U S A. 2005;102(44):15960–4.

37. Vulliamy TJ, Marrone A, Knight SW, et al. Mutations in dyskeratosis congenita: their impact on telomere length and the diversity of clinical presentation. Blood 2006;107(7):2680–5.

38. Feurstein S, Adegunsoye A, Mojsilovic D, et al. Telomere biology disorder prevalence and phenotypes in adults with familial hematologic and/or pulmonary presentations. Blood Adv 2020;4(19):4873–86.

39. Zhong F, Savage SA, Shkreli M, et al. Disruption of telomerase trafficking by TCAB1 mutation causes dyskeratosis congenita. Genes Dev 2011;25(1):11–6.

40. Vulliamy T, Beswick R, Kirwan M, et al. Mutations in the telomerase component NHP2 cause the premature ageing syndrome dyskeratosis congenita. Proc Natl Acad Sci U S A. 2008;105(23):8073–8.

41. Heiss NS, Knight SW, Vulliamy TJ, et al. X-linked dyskeratosis congenita is caused by mutations in a highly conserved gene with putative nucleolar functions. Nat Genet 1998;19(1):32–8.

42. Knight SW, Heiss NS, Vulliamy TJ, et al. X-linked dyskeratosis congenita is predominantly caused by missense mutations in the DKC1 gene. Am J Hum Genet 1999;65(1):50–8.

43. Richards LA, Kumari A, Knezevic K, et al. DKC1 is a transcriptional target of GATA1 and drives upregulation of telomerase activity in normal human erythroblasts. Haematologica 2020;105(6):1517–26.

44. Calado RT, Young NS. Telomere diseases. N Engl J Med 2009;361(24):2353–65.

45. Alter BP, Giri N, Savage SA, et al. Malignancies and survival patterns in the National Cancer Institute inherited bone marrow failure syndromes cohort study. Br J Haematol 2010;150(2):179–88.

46. Alter BP, Giri N, Savage SA, et al. Cancer in dyskeratosis congenita. Blood 2009; 113(26):6549–57.

47. Dokal I, Vulliamy T, Mason P, et al. Clinical utility gene card for: Dyskeratosis congenita - update 2015. Eur J Hum Genet 2015;23(4).

48. Alter BP, Baerlocher GM, Savage SA, et al. Very short telomere length by flow fluorescence in situ hybridization identifies patients with dyskeratosis congenita. Blood 2007;110(5):1439–47.
49. Tummala H, Walne A, Dokal I. The biology and management of dyskeratosis congenita and related disorders of telomeres. Expert Rev Hematol 2022; 15(8):685–96.
50. Elmahadi S, Muramatsu H, Kojima S. Allogeneic hematopoietic stem cell transplantation for dyskeratosis congenita. Curr Opin Hematol 2016;23(6):501–7.
51. Barbaro P, Vedi A. Survival after Hematopoietic Stem Cell Transplant in Patients with Dyskeratosis Congenita: Systematic Review of the Literature. Biol Blood Marrow Transplant 2016;22(7):1152–8.
52. Fioredda F, Iacobelli S, Korthof ET, et al. Outcome of haematopoietic stem cell transplantation in dyskeratosis congenita. Br J Haematol 2018;183(1):110–8.
53. Bagby GC, Alter BP. Fanconi anemia. Semin Hematol 2006;43(3):147–56.
54. Che R, Zhang J, Nepal M, et al. Multifaceted Fanconi Anemia Signaling. Trends Genet 2018;34(3):171–83.
55. Tipping AJ, Pearson T, Morgan NV, et al. Molecular and genealogical evidence for a founder effect in Fanconi anemia families of the Afrikaner population of South Africa. Proc Natl Acad Sci U S A 2001;98(10):5734–9.
56. Risitano AM, Marotta S, Calzone R, et al. Twenty years of the Italian Fanconi Anemia Registry: where we stand and what remains to be learned. Haematologica 2016;101(3):319–27.
57. Rosenberg PS, Tamary H, Alter BP. How high are carrier frequencies of rare recessive syndromes? Contemporary estimates for Fanconi Anemia in the United States and Israel. Am J Med Genet 2011;155A(8):1877–83.
58. Peake JD, Noguchi E. Fanconi anemia: current insights regarding epidemiology, cancer, and DNA repair. Hum Genet 2022;141(12):1811–36.
59. Dong H, Nebert DW, Bruford EA, et al. Update of the human and mouse Fanconi anemia genes. Hum Genomics 2015;9:32.
60. Faivre L, Guardiola P, Lewis C, et al. Association of complementation group and mutation type with clinical outcome in fanconi anemia. European Fanconi Anemia Research Group. Blood 2000;96(13):4064–70.
61. Alter BP. Fanconi anemia and the development of leukemia. Best Pract Res Clin Haematol 2014;27(3–4):214–21.
62. Alter BP, Giri N, Savage SA, et al. Cancer in the National Cancer Institute inherited bone marrow failure syndrome cohort after fifteen years of follow-up. Haematologica 2018;103(1):30–9.
63. Archibald H, Kalland K, Kuehne A, et al. Oral Premalignant and Malignant Lesions in Fanconi Anemia Patients. Laryngoscope 2023;133(7):1745–8.
64. Alter BP, Giri N. Thinking of VACTERL-H? Rule out Fanconi Anemia according to PHENOS. Am J Med Genet 2016;170(6):1520–4.
65. Oostra AB, Nieuwint AW, Joenje H, et al. Diagnosis of fanconi anemia: chromosomal breakage analysis. Anemia 2012;2012:238731.
66. Forlenza GP, Polgreen LE, Miller BS, et al. Growth hormone treatment of patients with Fanconi anemia after hematopoietic cell transplantation. Pediatr Blood Cancer 2014;61(6):1142–3.
67. Dufour C. How I manage patients with Fanconi anaemia. Br J Haematol 2017; 178(1):32–47.
68. Forastiere A, Koch W, Trotti A, et al. Head and neck cancer. N Engl J Med 2001; 345(26):1890–900.

69. Haddad RI, Shin DM. Recent advances in head and neck cancer. N Engl J Med 2008;359(11):1143–54.
70. Woo SB. Oral Epithelial Dysplasia and Premalignancy. Head Neck Pathol 2019; 13(3):423–39.
71. Warnakulasuriya S, Kujan O, Aguirre-Urizar JM, et al. Oral potentially malignant disorders: A consensus report from an international seminar on nomenclature and classification, convened by the WHO Collaborating Centre for Oral Cancer. Oral Dis 2021;27(8):1862–80.
72. Mello FW, Miguel AFP, Dutra KL, et al. Prevalence of oral potentially malignant disorders: A systematic review and meta-analysis. J Oral Pathol Med 2018; 47(7):633–40.
73. Iocca O, Sollecito TP, Alawi F, et al. Potentially malignant disorders of the oral cavity and oral dysplasia: A systematic review and meta-analysis of malignant transformation rate by subtype. Head Neck 2020;42(3):539–55.
74. Rao NR, Villa A, More CB, et al. Oral submucous fibrosis: a contemporary narrative review with a proposed inter-professional approach for an early diagnosis and clinical management. J Otolaryngol Head Neck Surg 2020;49(1):3.
75. Giuliani M, Troiano G, Cordaro M, et al. Rate of malignant transformation of oral lichen planus: A systematic review. Oral Dis 2019;25(3):693–709.
76. Lorenzo-Pouso AI, Lafuente-Ibanez de Mendoza I, Perez-Sayans M, et al. Critical update, systematic review, and meta-analysis of oral erythroplakia as an oral potentially malignant disorder. J Oral Pathol Med 2022;51(7):585–93.
77. Warnakulasuriya S, Johnson NW, van der Waal I. Nomenclature and classification of potentially malignant disorders of the oral mucosa. J Oral Pathol Med 2007;36(10):575–80.
78. Petti S. Pooled estimate of world leukoplakia prevalence: a systematic review. Oral Oncol 2003;39(8):770–80.
79. Villa A, Woo SB. Leukoplakia-A Diagnostic and Management Algorithm. J Oral Maxillofac Surg 2017;75(4):723–34.
80. Warnakulasuriya S. Clinical features and presentation of oral potentially malignant disorders. Oral Surg Oral Med Oral Pathol Oral Radiol 2018;125(6):582–90.
81. Villa A, Sonis S. Oral leukoplakia remains a challenging condition. Oral Dis 2018; 24(1–2):179–83.
82. Villa A, Menon RS, Kerr AR, et al. Proliferative leukoplakia: Proposed new clinical diagnostic criteria. Oral Dis 2018;24(5):749–60.
83. Pentenero M, Meleti M, Vescovi P, et al. Oral proliferative verrucous leucoplakia: are there particular features for such an ambiguous entity? A systematic review. Br J Dermatol 2014;170(5):1039–47.
84. Abadie WM, Partington EJ, Fowler CB, et al. Optimal Management of Proliferative Verrucous Leukoplakia: A Systematic Review of the Literature. Otolaryngol Head Neck Surg 2015;153(4):504–11.
85. Hanna GJ, Villa A, Mistry N, et al. Comprehensive Immunoprofiling of High-Risk Oral Proliferative and Localized Leukoplakia. Cancer Res Commun 2021;1(1): 30–40.
86. Kresty LA, Mallery SR, Knobloch TJ, et al. Alterations of p16(INK4a) and p14(ARF) in patients with severe oral epithelial dysplasia. Cancer Res 2002; 62(18):5295–300.
87. Okoturo EM, Risk JM, Schache AG, et al. Molecular pathogenesis of proliferative verrucous leukoplakia: a systematic review. Br J Oral Maxillofac Surg 2018; 56(9):780–5.

88. Warnakulasuriya S, Ariyawardana A. Malignant transformation of oral leukoplakia: a systematic review of observational studies. J Oral Pathol Med 2016; 45(3):155–66.
89. Ho MW, Risk JM, Woolgar JA, et al. The clinical determinants of malignant transformation in oral epithelial dysplasia. Oral Oncol 2012;48(10):969–76.
90. Lumerman H, Freedman P, Kerpel S. Oral epithelial dysplasia and the development of invasive squamous cell carcinoma. Oral Surg Oral Med Oral Pathol Oral Radiol Endod 1995;79(3):321–9.
91. Speight PM. Update on oral epithelial dysplasia and progression to cancer. Head Neck Pathol 2007;1(1):61–6.
92. Stojanov IJ, Woo SB. Malignant Transformation Rate of Non-reactive Oral Hyperkeratoses Suggests an Early Dysplastic Phenotype. Head Neck Pathol 2022; 16(2):366–74.
93. Monteiro L, Barbieri C, Warnakulasuriya S, et al. Type of surgical treatment and recurrence of oral leukoplakia: A retrospective clinical study. Med Oral Patol Oral Cir Bucal 2017;22(5):e520–6.
94. Kawczyk-Krupka A, Waskowska J, Raczkowska-Siostrzonek A, et al. Comparison of cryotherapy and photodynamic therapy in treatment of oral leukoplakia. Photodiagnosis Photodyn Ther 2012;9(2):148–55.
95. van der Hem PS, Nauta JM, van der Wal JE, et al. The results of CO_2 laser surgery in patients with oral leukoplakia: a 25 year follow up. Oral Oncol 2005; 41(1):31–7.
96. Liao YH, Chou WY, Chang CW, et al. Chemoprevention of oral cancer: A review and future perspectives. Head Neck 2023;45(4):1045–59.
97. de Pauli Paglioni M, Migliorati CA, Schausltz Pereira Faustino I, et al. Laser excision of oral leukoplakia: Does it affect recurrence and malignant transformation? A systematic review and meta-analysis. Oral Oncol 2020;109:104850.
98. Proano-Haro A, Bagan L, Bagan JV. Recurrences following treatment of proliferative verrucous leukoplakia: A systematic review and meta-analysis. J Oral Pathol Med 2021;50(8):820–8.
99. Mogedas-Vegara A, Hueto-Madrid JA, Chimenos-Kustner E, et al. Oral leukoplakia treatment with the carbon dioxide laser: A systematic review of the literature. J Cranio-Maxillo-Fac Surg 2016;44(4):331–6.
100. Palma VM, Koerich Laureano N, Frank LA, et al. Chemoprevention in oral leukoplakia: challenges and current landscape. Front Oral Health 2023;4:1191347.
101. Hanna GJ, Villa A, Nandi SP, et al. Nivolumab for Patients With High-Risk Oral Leukoplakia: A Nonrandomized Controlled Trial. JAMA Oncol 2024;10(1):32–41.
102. Silverman S Jr, Gorsky M, Lozada F. Oral leukoplakia and malignant transformation. A follow-up study of 257 patients. Cancer 1984;53(3):563–8.
103. Martinez VD, MacAulay CE, Guillaud M, et al. Targeting of chemoprevention to high-risk potentially malignant oral lesions: challenges and opportunities. Oral Oncol 2014;50(12):1123–30.
104. Califano J, van der Riet P, Westra W, et al. Genetic progression model for head and neck cancer: implications for field cancerization. Cancer Res 1996;56(11): 2488–92.
105. Mao L, Lee JS, Fan YH, et al. Frequent microsatellite alterations at chromosomes 9p21 and 3p14 in oral premalignant lesions and their value in cancer risk assessment. Nat Med 1996;2(6):682–5.
106. Zhang L, Poh CF, Williams M, et al. Loss of heterozygosity (LOH) profiles–validated risk predictors for progression to oral cancer. Cancer Prev Res 2012; 5(9):1081–9.

107. Rosin MP, Cheng X, Poh C, et al. Use of allelic loss to predict malignant risk for low-grade oral epithelial dysplasia. Clin Cancer Res 2000;6(2):357–62.
108. Rosin MP, Lam WL, Poh C, et al. 3p14 and 9p21 loss is a simple tool for predicting second oral malignancy at previously treated oral cancer sites. Cancer Res 2002;62(22):6447–50.
109. William WN Jr, Papadimitrakopoulou V, Lee JJ, et al. Erlotinib and the Risk of Oral Cancer: The Erlotinib Prevention of Oral Cancer (EPOC) Randomized Clinical Trial. JAMA Oncol 2016;2(2):209–16.
110. William WN Jr, Zhao X, Bianchi JJ, et al. Immune evasion in HPV(-) head and neck precancer-cancer transition is driven by an aneuploid switch involving chromosome 9p loss. Proc Natl Acad Sci U S A. 2021;118(19).
111. Datta M, Laronde DM, Rosin MP, et al. Predicting Progression of Low-Grade Oral Dysplasia Using Brushing-Based DNA Ploidy and Chromatin Organization Analysis. Cancer Prev Res 2021;14(12):1111–8.
112. William WN, Lee W-C, Lee JJ, et al. Genomic and transcriptomic landscape of oral pre-cancers (OPCs) and risk of oral cancer (OC). J Clin Oncol 2019; 37(15_suppl):6009.
113. Wils LJ, Poell JB, Brink A, et al. Elucidating the Genetic Landscape of Oral Leukoplakia to Predict Malignant Transformation. Clin Cancer Res 2023;29(3): 602–13.
114. Ohman J, Magnusson B, Telemo E, et al. Langerhans cells and T cells sense cell dysplasia in oral leukoplakias and oral squamous cell carcinomas–evidence for immunosurveillance. Scand J Immunol 2012;76(1):39–48.
115. Gannot G, Gannot I, Vered H, et al. Increase in immune cell infiltration with progression of oral epithelium from hyperkeratosis to dysplasia and carcinoma. Br J Cancer 2002;86(9):1444–8.
116. Ohman J, Mowjood R, Larsson L, et al. Presence of CD3-positive T-cells in oral premalignant leukoplakia indicates prevention of cancer transformation. Anticancer Res 2015;35(1):311–7.
117. Ries J, Agaimy A, Wehrhan F, et al. Importance of the PD-1/PD-L1 Axis for Malignant Transformation and Risk Assessment of Oral Leukoplakia. Biomedicines 2021;9(2).
118. Yagyuu T, Hatakeyama K, Imada M, et al. Programmed death ligand 1 (PD-L1) expression and tumor microenvironment: Implications for patients with oral precancerous lesions. Oral Oncol 2017;68:36–43.
119. William WN Jr, Zhang J, Zhao X, et al. Spatial PD-L1, immune-cell microenvironment, and genomic copy-number alteration patterns and drivers of invasive-disease transition in prospective oral precancer cohort. Cancer 2023;129(5): 714–27.
120. Khan MM, Frustino J, Villa A, et al. Total RNA sequencing reveals gene expression and microbial alterations shared by oral pre-malignant lesions and cancer. Hum Genomics 2023;17(1):72.
121. Zhao X, Cohen EEW, William WN Jr, et al. Somatic 9p24.1 alterations in HPV(-) head and neck squamous cancer dictate immune microenvironment and anti-PD-1 checkpoint inhibitor activity. Proc Natl Acad Sci U S A 2022;119(47): e2213835119.
122. Brennan M, Migliorati CA, Lockhart PB, et al. Management of oral epithelial dysplasia: a review. Oral Surg Oral Med Oral Pathol Oral Radiol Endod 2007; 103(Suppl):S19 e11–2.
123. William WN Jr. Oral premalignant lesions: any progress with systemic therapies? Curr Opin Oncol 2012;24(3):205–10.

124. Hittelman WN, Kim HJ, Lee JS, et al. Detection of chromosome instability of tissue fields at risk: in situ hybridization. J Cell Biochem Suppl 1996;25:57–62.

125. Monteiro de Oliveira Novaes JA, William WN Jr. Prognostic factors, predictive markers and cancer biology: the triad for successful oral cancer chemoprevention. Future Oncol 2016;12(20):2379–86.

126. Monteiro de Oliveira Novaes JA, Hirz T, Guijarro I, et al. Targeting of CD40 and PD-L1 Pathways Inhibits Progression of Oral Premalignant Lesions in a Carcinogen-induced Model of Oral Squamous Cell Carcinoma. Cancer Prev Res 2021;14(3):313–24.

127. Wang Z, Wu VH, Allevato MM, et al. Syngeneic animal models of tobacco-associated oral cancer reveal the activity of in situ anti-CTLA-4. Nat Commun 2019;10(1):5546.

128. Errazquin R, Page A, Sunol A, et al. Development of a mouse model for spontaneous oral squamous cell carcinoma in Fanconi anemia. Oral Oncol 2022; 134:106184.

129. Bouaoud J, Bossi P, Elkabets M, et al. Unmet Needs and Perspectives in Oral Cancer Prevention. Cancers 2022;14(7).

Ductal Carcinoma In Situ

Brittany L. Bychkovsky, MD, MSc[a,b,c], Sara Myers, MD, PhD[c,d],
Laura E.G. Warren, MD[c,e], Pietro De Placido, MD[b],
Heather A. Parsons, MD, MPH[b,c,f],*

KEYWORDS

- Ductal carcinoma in situ • DCIS • Breast cancer precursor lesions
- Breast cancer detection

KEY POINTS

- Ductal carcinoma in situ (DCIS) is a precancerous lesion of the breast and is most often detected after mammogram screening.
- Endocrine therapy has an established role in both primary and secondary prevention among females identified with DCIS or high-risk lesions who have intact breast tissue.
- Preliminary DCIS vaccine studies appear safe and can elicit sustained response, though further research is necessary to determine their clinical effectiveness.

BIOLOGY AND NATURAL CLINICAL HISTORY OF DUCTAL CARCINOMA IN SITU

In breast cancer (BC) pathogenesis models, normal cells acquire somatic mutations and there is a stepwise progression from high-risk lesions (HRLs include atypical ductal hyperplasia [ADH], atypical lobular hyperplasia [ALH], and lobular carcinoma in situ [LCIS]) and ductal carcinoma in situ (DCIS) to invasive cancer. The precancer biology of mammary tissue warrants better characterization to understand how different BC subtypes emerge. Currently, research efforts are underway to improve our understanding of premalignant biology and immunosurveillance in the precancer microenvironment to guide prevention and interception trials.[1,2]

DCIS is a precancerous lesion of the breast and is most often detected after mammogram screening. Microscopically, DCIS appears morphologically similar to invasive BCBC with uncontrolled proliferation of neoplastic cells that obliterate the normal lobular and ductal structures; however, unlike invasive BCBC, DCIS does not invade across the basement membrane.[3]

a Division of Cancer Genetics and Prevention, Dana-Farber Cancer Institute, Boston, MA, USA; b Department of Medical Oncology, Dana-Farber Cancer Institute, Boston, MA, USA; c Harvard Medical School, Boston, MA, USA; d Brigham and Women's Hospital, Boston, MA, USA; e Department of Radiation Oncology, Dana-Farber Cancer Institute, Boston, MA, USA; f Broad Institute of MIT and Harvard, Cambridge, MA, USA
* Corresponding author. Dana-Farber Cancer Institute, 450 Brookline Avenue, Boston, MA 02115.
E-mail address: heather_parsons@dfci.harvard.edu

Hematol Oncol Clin N Am 38 (2024) 831–849
https://doi.org/10.1016/j.hoc.2024.05.014
0889-8588/24/© 2024 Elsevier Inc. All rights reserved.

At diagnosis, the estrogen receptor (ER) status of DCIS is determined as this influences recommendations for endocrine therapy (and radiation therapy [RT] among older patients). Tamoxifen or an aromatase inhibitor (AI) can reduce the risk of recurrence and a second BCBC diagnosis.[4–10] Increased expression of ER distinguishes precancer lesions from normal breast tissue, and is an important regulator of BC pathogenesis.[11] In contrast, ER-negative DCIS is perceived as a more aggressive phenotype and is seen more frequently in palpable DCIS versus asymptomatic screen-detected DCIS[12]; however, this perception may be influenced by the fact that there are no established preventative systemic therapies for ER-negative DCIS at this time.

High-grade DCIS with comedonecrosis is associated with an increased risk of invasive disease,[13,14] ipsilateral disease recurrence,[15] and tumor-infiltrating lymphocytes (TILs).[3] A high number of TILs and the distribution of TILs in the DCIS microenvironment are correlated with DCIS outcomes.[16] TILs in DCIS are associated with somatic TP53 mutations, which are more common with ER-negative HER2-positive DCIS, and higher nuclear grade.[3] Prior work has also demonstrated that the immune microenvironment differs between DCIS alone, DCIS with microinvasion, and invasive BC, and these differences can be further stratified by ER status.[17] In sum, at least a subset of DCIS is immunogenic and therefore, vaccination or immunomodulatory therapies may have a role in BC prevention and risk-reduction for patients with DCIS or HRLs.

PRIMARY AND SECONDARY PREVENTION

Endocrine therapy has an established role in both primary and secondary prevention among females identified with DCIS or an HRL who have intact breast tissue. Premenopausal females are eligible for tamoxifen 20 mg, and postmenopausal females are eligible for tamoxifen 20 mg, tamoxifen 5 mg, raloxifene, exemestane, or anastrozole. The approach to endocrine therapy in this patient population is evolving due new data showing good efficacy of low-dose tamoxifen for prevention and risk-reduction.[9,10]

The impact of tamoxifen 20 mg/d for a duration of 5 years (compared to placebo) was examined among patients with DCIS who had received a breast conservation surgery (BCS) and radiation in the National Surgery Adjuvant Breast and Bowel Project (NSABP) B-24 (A Clinical Trial to Evaluate the Worth of Tamoxifen in Conjunction with Lumpectomy and Breast Irradiation for the Treatment of Noninvasive Intraductal Carcinoma (DCIS) of the Breast) study.[4] ER testing was not required for study enrollment, but was available for 41% of the cohort. On subset analyses, tamoxifen 20 mg/d for 5 years was found to reduce the rates of any subsequent DCIS or invasive cancer event among patients with ER-positive DCIS (hazard ratio [HR] 0.58; 95% confidence interval [CI]: 0.415–0.81; $P=.0015$), but not in those with ER-negative DCIS (HR 0.88; 95% CI: 0.49–1.59; $P=.68$). For those with ER-positive DCIS, the benefit was primarily due to a statistically significant reduction in contralateral BC (CBC) events (HR 0.50; 95% CI: 0.28–0.88; $P<.02$). Statistical significance was not reached for ipsilateral breast events (HR 0.68; 95% CI: 0.44–1.03; $P<.07$) demonstrating that the primary benefit of tamoxifen is to reduce the risk of future CBCs. For those with ER-negative DCIS, tamoxifen 20 mg for 5 years did not have a statistically significant benefit at reducing any future BC diagnosis, ipsilateral BC, or CBC; however, the event rate was low for CBC with 7 CBCs in those that received placebo and 3 among those who received tamoxifen.[4] Among those with invasive disease, ER status is not necessarily predictive of the BC subtype that may emerge when a patient develops a second BC: among females with ER-negative invasive BC who develop a second BC, ER concordance occurs 53% of the time and among females with ER-positive invasive BC who develop a second BC, ER concordance is 82%.[18]

Tamoxifen 20 mg for 5 years also has efficacy for primary prevention. In the NSABP P-1 (A Clinical Trial to Determine the Worth of Tamoxifen for Preventing Breast Cancer) trial,[5] premenopausal or postmenopausal females aged more than 60, or females aged 35 to 60 at elevated risk for BC as defined by the presence of an HRL (ADH, ALH, LCIS) or a Gail 5-year risk score of $\geq$ 1.67, were randomized to tamoxifen 20 mg/day for 5 years (n = 6597) or placebo (n = 6610).[5] At 7 years of follow-up, tamoxifen reduced the risk of invasive BC (rate ratio[RR] 0.57; 95% CI: 0.46–0.70) and noninvasive disease (DCIS) compared to placebo (RR 0.63; 95% CI: 0.45–0.89).[5] Tamoxifen also had a benefit of reducing osteoporotic fractures by 32%, but did increase the risk of endometrial cancer, primarily in females aged 50 and older (RR 5.33; 95% CI: 2.47–13.17) compared to those aged 49 or younger (RR 1.42; 95% CI: 0.55–3.81).[5] The cumulative risk of endometrial cancer at 7 years of follow-up was 0.468% in the placebo group and 1.5% with tamoxifen (P<.001)[5]; importantly, all were early-stage cancers and were treated with simple hysterectomy. Tamoxifen 20 mg also statistically increased the risk of pulmonary embolism (PE) (0.69 per 1000 for tam vs 0.32 per 1000 for placebo, RR 2.15; 95% CI: 1.08–4.51), and there was a trend toward an increased risk of deep vein thrombosis (DVT) (1.21 per 1000 for tamoxifen vs 0.84 per 1000 for placebo, RR 1.44; 95% CI: 0.91–2.3).[5]

Subsequent to the NSABP P-1 study, 3 additional trials demonstrated that tamoxifen 20 mg for 5 years reduces the risk of BC.[6–8] In the IBIS-1 (Tamoxifen for the Prevention of Breast Cancer in High-Risk Women) study, females were followed for a median of 16.0 years and it was demonstrated that 5 years of endocrine therapy with tamoxifen has a long-lasting effect on risk reduction.[6] The risk reduction of developing BC with tamoxifen 20 mg for 5 years was similar between years 0 to 10 (HR 0.72; 95% CI: 0.59–0.88, P=.001) and after 10 years (HR 0.69; 95% CI: 0.53–0.91, P=.009).[6]

After 2 studies found that a subset of older patients with ER-positive DCIS could avoid adjuvant radiation without an increased risk of ipsilateral recurrence if they received adjuvant endocrine therapy,[19,20] 2 randomized control trials were conducted comparing tamoxifen to an AI: IBIS-II DCIS (An International Multi-Centre Trial of Tamoxifen Versus Anastrozole in Postmenopausal Women who have had a Recent Hormone Receptor Positive Ductal Carcinoma In Situ) and NSABP B-35 (Anastrozole or Tamoxifen in Treating Postmenopausal Women With Ductal Carcinoma in Situ Who Are Undergoing Lumpectomy and Radiation Therapy).[21,22] In the IBIS-II DCIS study,[21] there was no difference in recurrence rates at median follow-up of 7.2 years for patients who received anastrozole versus tamoxifen (HR 0.89; 95% CI: 0.64–1.23). In IBIS-II DCIS, 71% received radiation and this was balanced between the 2 arms.[21] NSABP B-35 was also a randomized controlled trial comparing tamoxifen 20 mg to anastrozole; however, all participants received radiation.[22] In contrast, NSABP B-35 showed that anastrozole reduced the risk of all breast events (HR 0.73; 95% CI: 0.56–0.96; P=.02) and contralateral breast events (HR 0.64; 95% CI: 0.43–0.96; P=.03) compared to tamoxifen.[22] The benefit was limited to postmenopausal females aged less than 60 compared to those aged 60 and older, which is noteworthy as women often have more musculoskeletal problems and bone loss as they age. In IBIS-II DCIS, there were higher rates of musculoskeletal side effects (64% with anastrozole vs 54% with tamoxifen) and fractures (9% vs 7%) with AI therapy compared to tamoxifen.[21] At this time in clinical practice, AIs are available for prevention among those with DCIS or HRLs of the breast, and the recommended approach must consider patient preferences and the risks of therapy.

Recent work has suggested that measurement of serum estradiol and testosterone levels could guide care decisions among postmenopausal patients on an AI for prevention. At a median follow-up of $\sim$10 years, the IBIS-II (Anastrozole in Preventing

Breast Cancer in Postmenopausal Women at Increased Risk of Breast Cancer) prevention trial found a benefit to anastrozole among patients with estradiol/sex hormone binding globulin ratios of ≥ 0.167,[23] but less relative benefit when ratio was less than 0.167 (relative benefit 0.18; 95% CI: -0.60–0.59). These findings suggest that biomarker monitoring could inform clinical care.

Despite the known benefit of endocrine therapy in primary and secondary prevention for women with a diagnosis of DCIS, many do not start or are unable to tolerate AI or tamoxifen due to adverse effects.[24–26] Approaches to maintain the benefits but avoid toxicity may help with endocrine therapy uptake. More recently, there is robust data supporting low-dose tamoxifen for primary and secondary prevention among females who are high risk or have a personal diagnosis of DCIS. In TAM-01 (Trial of Low Dose Tamoxifen in Women With Breast Intraepithelial Neoplasia - Long Term Follow-up) trial, low-dose tamoxifen 5 mg was compared to placebo, and included 500 women with a diagnosis of DCIS, ADH, or LCIS who received breast conservation therapy.[9] Most patients in the study had a diagnosis of DCIS (69% in the low-dose tamoxifen arm and 70% in the placebo arm; yet ER status was only known in 80% of cases with DCIS and only 45% of patients received RT). At a median follow-up of 9.7 years,[10] there was a benefit to low-dose tamoxifen: 9.8% in the tamoxifen 5 mg arm were diagnosed with BC compared to 16.6% who were in the placebo group (HR 0.58; 95% CI: 0.35–0.95, $P=.03$).[10] Most recurrences were invasive (77%) and ipsilateral (59%).[10] Regarding the CBC rate, there were 6 BCs with tamoxifen 5 mg and 16 with placebo (HR 0.36; 95% CI: 0.14–0.92, $P=.025$).[10] Within subgroup analyses, patients with DCIS had a 50% reduction in BC recurrence with low-dose tamoxifen for 3 years (HR 0.50; 95% CI: 0.28–0.91, $P=.02$). The reduction in BC events occurred while patients were on tamoxifen 5 mg for 3 years and were durable for 7 years after therapy cessation demonstrating a role for low-dose tamoxifen for primary and secondary prevention.

Low-dose tamoxifen has an exceptional side effect profile.[10] In TAM-01, there were no differences in rates of DVT/PE, coronary heart disease, bone fracture, cataract, endometrial polyps, and endometrial cancer rates between patients who received low-dose tamoxifen for 3 years versus those who received placebo. There are more hot flashes with tamoxifen 5 mg compared to placebo ($P=.02$); this effectively translated into 1 more hot flash per day.[9] There were no differences between hot flash intensity ($P=.16$), vaginal dryness ($P=.40$), or musculoskeletal pain or arthralgias ($P=.41$) between the 2 study arms.

Subset analyses of TAM-01 showed that postmenopausal females, with estradiol less than 15.8 pg/mL, menopausal symptoms at baseline, and those who were never smokers benefited most from low-dose tamoxifen.[27] Among postmenopausal women, low-dose tamoxifen had a favorable HR (HR = 0.30; 95% CI: 0.11–0.82) compared to premenopausal women (HR = 0.73; 95% CI: 0.30–1.76) and this was borderline statistically significant $P_{interaction} = 0.13$. More work is needed to better understand if low levels of active tamoxifen metabolites (with low-dose tamoxifen) are less effective in premenopausal women compared to postmenopausal women due to the higher baseline levels of estrogen in premenopausal women. Body mass index (BMI) did not influence tamoxifen 5 mg efficacy,[27] which is consistent with prior work that efficacy of tamoxifen 20 mg is not influence by BMI.[28,29] This finding is similar to what has been observed with AIs where BMI is not a modulating factor of outcome in the prevention setting.[30]

Patients with baseline menopausal symptoms are unlikely to take either selective estrogen receptor modulators (SERMs) or an AI, and ongoing work is investigating bazedoxifene combined with conjugated estrogen (CE) (BZE + CE, Duavee) in the prevention setting. Preclinical data suggest that BZE + CE downregulates ERalpha and Ki67 expression similar to BZE alone and distinct from CE, and therefore may have a role for BC prevention.[31] Ongoing work has demonstrated that BZE can induce epigenetic changes in 17beta-estradiol (E2) and other estrogen compounds that mediate ERalpha regulator changes to target gene proliferative pathways.[32] Clinical data are also promising showing favorable effects on BC risk biomarkers when women were treated for 6 months with BZE + CE,[33] and a phase II trial is ongoing (NCT04821141).

At this time, there is a need to better understand the immunomodulatory effects of SERMs and AI in the prevention setting since our understanding of anticancer immunity and the breast microenvironment has evolved since these agents were first studied.[34,35] It is unclear if there are different immunologic effects between SERMs and AIs that could be combined synergically with novel therapies to enhance BC prevention among those with HRLs and DCIS.

SURGICAL CONSIDERATIONS

Surgery is the mainstay of treatment for DCIS.[36] The National Comprehensive Cancer Network treatment guidelines indicate that appropriate candidates may be offered either BCS or mastectomy.[37] Traditionally, contraindications to BCS for DCIS included extensive disease,[38] multicentricity, and multifocality.[39] It is estimated that for unilateral DCIS, 70% of women receive BCS compared to 20% who undergo unilateral mastectomy; bilateral mastectomy is pursued by 10% of women.[40]

Local recurrence varies by surgical approach: compared to the 1% to 2% local recurrence rate after mastectomy, recurrence after BCS depends on tumor characteristics, margin status, receipt of endocrine (ER+) and radiation treatments in the adjuvant setting.[41] In patients $\geq$ 40 years old who receive BCS for unifocal DCIS followed by radiation, society guidelines advocate for a margin of at least 2 mm to minimize the risk of local recurrence.[42] Optimal margin width in younger patients with large or multifocal disease is unclear based on existing data. The Memorial Sloan Kettering Cancer Center has a freely available prognostic nomogram to assist in understanding DCIS recurrence rates after BCS allowing for individualized approach to adjuvant treatment (ie, radiation and/or endocrine therapy).[43] Other prediction tools that aid in understanding recurrence and may be used to guide shared decision-making with respect to choice of surgical treatment include the Oncotype DX DCIS Score[44] and DCISionRT Prelude DX.[20] Discussion of how these tools can be leveraged for decisions to pursue adjuvant radiation and endocrine therapy will be discussed elsewhere.

Axillary staging is not generally recommended for patients undergoing BCS. There is variability in surgeon practice; however, with data from the National Cancer Database indicating that 19% of patients undergoing BCS for DCIS receive sentinel lymph node biopsy (SLNB).[45] Features such as tumor size greater than 3 cm, high histologic grade, and necrosis may motivate some to pursue SLNB[46] despite the low probability of pathologic node positivity. Studies advocating for the omission of SLNB include a meta-analysis of 9803 patients from 48 studies that demonstrated safety in patients with high-grade DCIS smaller than 2 cm and low to intermediate grade DCIS over 2 cm.[47] A Surveillance, Epidemiology, and End Results population database analysis corroborated these findings in patients 67 years of age or older in who there were no differences in locoregional recurrence or survival based on receipt of SLNB.[48] In the case of mastectomy, SLNB is usually performed given concern that postoperative assessment in the setting of upstage to invasive carcinoma would be compromised after removal of the breast.

Existing data indicate that only 20% to 30% of DCIS progresses to invasive ductal carcinoma (IDC).[49,50] Unfortunately, factors that confer risk of progression are incompletely understood.[51] As such, clinical trials are underway investigating whether surveillance is a safe alternative to operative management.[52–55] Forthcoming data from these trials will be helpful in deciphering a subpopulation of patients who may be surveilled with or without endocrine therapy in lieu of surgical resection (**Tables 1 and 2**).

Radiation

Several studies dating back to the 1980s to 1990s examined the benefit of RT following BCS for DCIS. A meta-analysis of 3729 patients from 4 trials—NSABP B-17 (A Protocol to Evaluate Natural History and Treatment of Patients with Noninvasive Intraductal Adenocarcinoma), EORTC 10853, SweDCIS (Swedish Breast Cancer Group Ductal Carcinoma in Situ), and UK ANZ DCIS (UK, Australia, and New Zealand Ductal Carcinoma In Situ)—randomizing patients to RT or not following BCS showed that RT approximately halved the rate of ipsilateral breast events (RR, 0.46; standard error (SE) 0.05; $P<.00001$) with an absolute benefit of 15.2% at 10 years.[56] RT was beneficial regardless of other risk factors including age, grade, pathologic size, extent of BCS, whether tamoxifen was planned, and whether or not comedonecrosis was present. Investigators defined a lower risk subgroup as patients with negative margins and low-grade DCIS measuring 1 to 20 mm, and RT still proved beneficial in lowering the 10-year risk of an ipsilateral event from 30.1% to 12.1% (RR, 0.48; SE 0.17; $P = .002$). Despite the substantial reduction in recurrence, there was no difference in BC mortality or overall survival, likely due to the success of salvage therapy in the event of a recurrence. These data provided strong support for the routine use of adjuvant RT for patients with DCIS, irrespective of clinical or pathologic features, as a means by which to decrease the risk of in-breast recurrence (IBR) following BCS.

However, patients treated for DCIS in the modern era have a lower absolute risk of IBR, likely due to of a combination of increased mammographic screening, improved imaging quality and pathologic evaluation, and increased utilization of adjuvant RT and endocrine therapy. Recent efforts have focused on better identifying a low-risk subgroup of patients who might safely avoid RT. The Eastern Cooperative Oncology Group-American College of Radiology Imaging Network (ECOG-ACRIN) trial E5194 (Evaluation of Breast Cancer Recurrence Rates Following Surgery in Women With Ductal Carcinoma In Situ) enrolled 2 cohorts of patients with DCIS to evaluate omission of RT: (1)lLow-grade or intermediate-grade DCIS measuring 2.5 cm or smaller (n = 561) or (2) high-grade DCIS measuring 1 cm or smaller (n = 104).[20] Surgical margins were 3 mm or greater. The 12-year rate of an ipsilateral local recurrence was 14.4% and 24.6% in cohorts 1 and 2, respectively, and continued to increase over the follow-up period without plateau. For patients with high-grade DCIS, these data are often referenced in support of a recommendation for adjuvant RT given the high risk of local recurrence with the omission of RT.

The Radiation Therapy Oncology Group 9804 (Radiation Therapy With or Without Optional Tamoxifen in Treating Women With Ductal Carcinoma in Situ) trial similarly attempted to identify a group of patients at low risk of IBR who may be candidates for omission of RT. This was a randomized, prospective trial of 636 patients with good-risk DCIS, defined as mammographically detected, low-grade or intermediate-grade DCIS, measuring 2.5 cm or less with margins 3 mm or greater. Patients meeting these criteria were randomized to RT or observation after BCS. Of the enrolled patients, 76% were postmenopausal, 44% had grade 1 DCIS, the median pathologic size was 0.6 cm, and 65% had margins ≥1.0 cm. At a median follow-up time of 7.2 years, RT decreased the 7-year risk of local failure from 6.7% (95% CI, 3.2%–9.6%) to 0.9%

Table 1
Trials of active surveillance for ductal carcinoma in situ

	LOw RISk DCIS (LORIS) Trial	Comparison of Operative versus Monitoring and Endocrine Therapy (COMET) Trial	The Low Risk DCIS (LORD) Trial
Study design	RCT	RCT	RCT
Primary endpoint	5 y—ipsilateral invasive breast cancer–free survival	2–5 y ipsilateral invasive cancer diagnosis	10 y ipsilateral invasive breast cancer and cancer-free survival
Inclusion criteria	≥ 46 y with a histologically confirmed diagnosis of grade I/II DCIS	≥ 46 y with any extent of ER/PR + grade I/II DCIS who had confirmed diagnosis based on biopsy or lumpectomy (positive margins allowed) ≤120 d of registration	≥ 45 y with any extent of grade I/II DCIS
Exclusion criteria	• Previous ipsilateral DCIS or invasive breast cancer • Mass lesion not biopsy-proven benign • High-risk group for developing breast cancer • Comedonecrosis	• Previous history of DCIS or invasive breast cancer • HER2 + disease	• Previous history of DCIS or invasive breast cancer • Family history of BRCA 1/2 mutation • Symptomatic DCIS
Imaging schedule	Annual bilateral mammography	Ipsilateral mammography every 6 m; Contralateral mammography annually	Annual bilateral mammography
Endocrine therapy	Optional	Optional	Not allowed

Abbreviations: DCIS, ductal carcinoma in situ; ER, estrogen receptor; HER2, human epidermal growth factor 2; PR, progesterone receptor; RCT, randomized controlled trial.

Adapted from Hwang ES, Malek V. Estimating the magnitude of clinical benefit of local therapy in patients with DCIS. Breast. Nov 2019;48 Suppl 1:S34-S38. (https://doi.org/10.1016/S0960-9776193110-8)

Table 2
Overview of prediction models predicting subsequence breast events after ductal carcinoma in situ

	Oncotype DCIS (Solin et al,[61] 2013)	DCISionRT PreludeDX (Bremer et al,[44] 2018)	Van Nuys Prognostic Index (Silverstein et al, 1995)	MSKCC DCIS Nomogram (Rudlof et al,[43] 2010)	Patient Prognostic Score (Sagara et al, 2016)	CBC Risk Model (Choudhury et al, 2017)
Country	USA	Sweden	USA	USA	USA	USA
Format	On order*	On order**	On paper	Web-based***	On paper	On paper
Predicted outcome	Ipsilateral in situ or invasive breast event	Ipsilateral in situ or invasive breast event	Disease-free survival	Ipsilateral in situ or invasive breast event	Breast cancer–specific death	Contralateral invasive breast cancer
Tool based on	Multigene assay	Clinicopathological factors	Clinicopathological factors	Clinicopathological factors	Clinicopathological factors	Clinicopathological factors
Type of data	Trial cohort	Multicenter	Single-center	Trial cohort	Population-based	Population-based
Number of patients	327	526	238	1868	32,144	7,684
Number of events	46	Not reported	31	202	304	1,921
Intended to support decision making about:	Adjuvant radiotherapy	Adjuvant radiotherapy	Type of surgery and adjuvant radiotherapy	Adjuvant radiotherapy	Adjuvant radiotherapy	Screening or prophylactic mastectomy
Risk of bias based on CHARMS	Moderate	Moderate	Moderate/high	Moderate	Moderate	Moderate
Number of validation studies retrieved	3	2	10	3	0	0

Type of data validation studies	Trial and population-based	Trial and single center	Single-center and Multicenter	Single-center	N.A.	N.A.
Number of patients validation studies (range)	718–1102	455–504	159–949	467–734	N.A.	N.A.
Number of events validation studies (range)	65–100	54–90	11–165	42–63	N.A.	N.A.
C-index/AUC	0.68	None reported	None reported	0.61–0.68	None reported	None reported
Clinical utility	Unclear	Unclear	Unclear	Unclear	Unclear	Unclear

Adapted from Dabbs D, Mittal K, Heineman S, Whitworth P, Shah C, Savala J, Shivers SC and Bremer T (2023) Analytical validation of the 7-gene biosignature for prediction of recurrence risk and radiation therapy benefit for breast ductal carcinoma in situ. Front. Oncol. 13:1069059. https://doi.org/10.3389/fonc.2023.1069059.

(95% CI, 0.0% to 2.2%); HR 0.11 (95% CI, 0.03–0.47; P<.001).[57] Long-term follow-up demonstrated a persistent reduction in IBR with the utilization of RT; 15-year IBR decreased from 15.1% (95% CI, 10.8–20.2) to 7.1% (95% CI, 4.0–11.5) with the addition of RT (HR = 0.36; 95% CI, 0.20–0.66; P = .0007).[58] There was no significant difference in subsequent mastectomy rates between treatment arms and no difference in overall survival. These data demonstrate that the risk of IBR continues to increase over time, particularly after 10 years of follow-up, and that adjuvant RT significantly decreases this risk. Specifically, and importantly, these studies demonstrate a reduction in the risk of both in situ and invasive recurrences with the utilization of RT.

In the hopes of better quantifying and personalizing estimates of the risk of IBR and the benefits of adjuvant RT for patients with DCIS, multigene molecular profiling assays have been developed. The Oncotype DX DCIS Score (Genomic Health) is a 12-gene prognostic test that was developed to estimate the 10-year risk of IBR following BCS alone. Its prognostic value was initially validated in a cohort of over 3000 women with DCIS[59] and it was subsequently shown to be predictive of the benefit of RT.[60] All patients benefited from RT but those with a higher score derived a greater absolute benefit from RT compared to those with lower scores, approximately 13% versus 5% absolute risk reduction in the modern era, respectively. Oncotype DX DCIS score was calculated for a subset of patients from the ECOG-ACRIN 5194 study (n = 327) and was found to be significantly associated with local control at 10 years, independent of other traditional clinical and pathologic features.[61] Despite enrollment eligibility based on perceived lower risk features, 30% of patients enrolled on ECOG-ACRIN 5194 were categorized into the intermediate-risk or high-risk groups based on their DCIS score. The DUCHESS (Evaluation of the DCIS Score for Decisions on Radiotherapy in Patients With Low/Intermediate Risk DCIS) trial attempted to assess the impact of the DCIS score, in conjunction with traditional clinical-pathologic features, on the recommendation for RT in a cohort of 217 patients. The score changed the treatment recommendation in 35.2% (95% CI, 29.1%–41.8%) of patients, improved patient satisfaction, and reduced decisional conflict.[62]

DCISionRT (Prelude Dx) is a genomic assay that risk stratifies patients into low and elevated risk based on data from 7 genes and 4 clinical-pathologic factors. On multivariate analysis, DCISionRT was independently associated with 10-year IBR.[44] Patients defined as low risk by DCISionRT had similar IBR with or without RT; the elevated risk group had significantly decreased rates of IBR with the receipt of RT (HR, 0.3; P = .003). The PREDICT (The PREDICT Registry for DCIS Patients With DCISionRT Testing) study is a prospective cohort study that is evaluating the effect of DCISionRT on treatment recommendations for patients with DCIS following BCS. DCISionRT testing resulted in a substantial change in RT recommendations with 42% of recommendations changing after receipt of the score and overall adjuvant RT being recommended in 20% fewer patients.[63] Although additional data are forthcoming, there are to date no randomized data supporting routine incorporation of molecular profiling to guide recommendations for adjuvant RT and the cost-effectiveness of this testing should also be considered before widespread adoption.[64]

In conclusion, prospective trials have demonstrated that even in patients with DCIS felt to be at low risk for IBR following BCS, the risk of IBR increases with time and adjuvant RT lowers this risk. RT does not, however, confer an overall survival benefit. While adjuvant RT has been shown to decrease the risk of IBR, there are potential side effects including radiation dermatitis and fatigue in the acute setting and breast discomfort, skin color changes, and, modest but non-zero, risks of RT-related pneumonitis, ischemic heart disease, and secondary malignancy in the longer term. While increasing utilization of shorter, hypofractionated courses of radiation decreases the risk of financial toxicity that is another potential consideration when deciding to proceed with adjuvant RT.[65] Therefore, for many patients, whether to proceed with adjuvant RT is a shared decision informed by the patient's perceived value of the decreased risk of IBR weighed against the potential side effects.

Future Approaches in Detection and Risk Stratification

Given the high incidence and local recurrence rate of DCIS, future research efforts are vital in this field. Priority areas include (a) enhancing early detection through novel body fluid biomarkers; (b) refining risk stratification according to genetics, radiological, and clinical features; and (c) preventive interventions incorporating immunomodulation via vaccines.

EARLY DETECTION

Current approaches to DCIS detection rely on mammography. Successful advancements in early detection should enable increased DCIS diagnoses, while also differentiating between high-risk and low-risk cases. If successful, this would allow for a reduction in the number of tumors presenting as IDC and for treatment tailoring across risk scenarios. This goal might be achieved via newly emerging technologies to detect blood-based biomarkers with recent investigations illustrating the current strengths and limitations of this approach.

Progress in genomics, sequencing, and machine learning have facilitated the development of blood tests for cancer detection, monitoring, and selecting treatment.[66–72] These technologies rely on detection of circulating nucleic acids, usually cell-free DNA (cfDNA) released by precancerous cells, or circulating tumor DNA (ctDNA). Initial studies investigating early detection of DCIS and invasive BC have been limited by test sensitivity. In a study conducted in Japan using the Oncomine Pan-Cancer cell-free assay to detect ctDNA, 1/12 (8%) patients with stage 0 disease, out of a cohort of 109 with early and metastatic BC (BC), were identified by the assay.[73] The PATHFINDER study (NCT04241796) is an excellent example of scientific progress in this field using a multi-cancer early detection (MCED) test based on cancer-specific DNA methylation patterns from cfDNA. The test can detect a cancer signal and predict the origin discriminating more than 50 distinct cancer types.[68,70] Results show a cancer signal detected in 92/6621 pan-cancer participants, anticipating the diagnosis in 35 confirmed to be true positives,[74] and demonstrating the feasibility of MCED testing in screening. However, performance in BC was limited. Results are awaited from newly designed trials: The PATHFINDER2 cohort study (NCT05155605), the UK's NHS Galleri study (ISRCTN91431511),[75] and the Oxford's SYMPLIFY study (ISRCTN10226380),[76] all evaluating the MCED testing as a screening procedure.

Some assays instead rely on the detection of molecular profiles of microRNA (miRNA). Shimomura and colleagues[77] examined 5 miRNA expression profiles in the serum of both BC patients and healthy women, demonstrating a sensitivity of 98.0% with DCIS. The authors are now working on moving this into prospective clinical studies. Early detection is key to achieve better outcomes in early-stage cancers such as DCIS and further advancements are required in diagnostic tools to enhance affordability, speed, and ease of use. Future combined approaches could improve analytical sensitivity of screening procedures through detection of ctDNA and circulating tumor cells in plasma or urine.

RISK STRATIFICATION AND TREATMENT TAILORING STRATEGIES

To optimize therapeutic strategies, risk stratification is essential and includes understanding patients' intrinsic predisposition, and radiological and clinical features.

Risk-stratified prevention programs are typically evaluated in randomized trials or prospective studies integrating data from screening for inherited pathogenic variants in high-risk genes, along with tumor radiological characteristics, and disease clinical features, all constituting factors which dynamically interact over time. Such studies take a long time to be finalized and simulation models can complement trial results.[78–82]

Evidence of DCIS sharing the same genetic predisposition with IDC come from a UK's King College study in which data pooled from 38 studies with a total of 5067 cases of DCIS, 24,584 cases of IDC and nearly 38,000 controls, all genotyped using a custom Illumina iSelect genotyping array, designed as part of the Collaborative Oncological Gene-Environment Study (iCOGS chip) showed no significant difference analyzing the 76 known BC predisposition loci.[83]

Conventional radiology can serve as a backbone diagnostic to be complemented by additional testing. Dynamic contrast-enhanced breast MRI is the most sensitive imaging to detect and characterize DCIS.[84] A small MRI radiomics study showed that heterogeneity features could differentiate DCIS nuclear grades.[85] The artificial intelligence may bridge radiomics and DCIS management in the future. In a pilot study, semiquantitative MRI features could discriminate DCIS nuclear grades and identify low-risk DCIS based on the Van Nuys score.[86,87]

DCIS evaluation with contrast-enhanced mammography (CEM) is still challenging, even though proven to be non-inferior to MRI in less than 5-mm lesions[88,89]; from retrospective evidence, CEM shows high sensitivity, suggesting that the enhancement may correlate with nuclear grade.[90,91]

With around 20% to 30% progressing to invasive BC if left untreated, DCIS management needs focused-research interventions.[92,93] This indicates that much of the treatment provided may be overtreatment. Low-risk DCIS has emerged as a distinct subtype that could potentially be managed with active surveillance (AS), as some patients will never develop invasive BC.[53,94,95]

The COMET trial (NCT02926911) is a currently ongoing phase III randomized controlled clinical trial for low-risk DCIS designed with a specific objective: to determine the risks and benefits of guideline concordant care (GCC) compared with those of AS for low-risk DCIS. In this study, low-risk disease is defined as 40 years of age or older, grade I/II DCIS without invasive BC diagnosed on biopsy; ER+ and/or progesterone receptor+; HER2-; and no mass on physical examination or imaging.[53] In addition, The LOw Risk dcIS study (LORIS trial; ISRCTN27544579) is a randomized controlled trial of AS versus GCC in the UK, which opened to accrual in 2015.[52] The principal investigators of the LORIS study collaborated with the COMET study team to coordinate studies endpoints, facilitating future meta-analysis.[53]

Multidisciplinary collaboration, intrinsic predisposition, and advanced imaging techniques play crucial roles in guiding treatment decisions and addressing the challenges associated with DCIS.

Future directions in treatment: vaccination

Currently, primary methods for BC prevention or risk reduction include lifestyle changes, surgery, and chemoprevention. Surgical intervention for BC prevention involves risk-reducing prophylactic mastectomy, typically performed either synchronously with the treatment of a primary tumor or as a bilateral procedure in high-risk women. Chemoprevention with endocrine therapy carries adherence-limiting toxicity. New, effective strategies for BC prevention are an unmet need, and cancer vaccines represent a promising potential approach.

Cancer immunosurveillance is critical for interception and elimination of evolving neoplastic cells.[96] High CD8 + T cells concentration in a tumor and adjacent stroma is associated with improved BC prognosis, indicating that malignant cells have been identified and an immune response elicited.[97] BC vaccines are a developing approach leveraging the host immune system to offer defense against cancer, preventing the advancement of HRLs to invasive ones. Studies of dendritic cell (DC) vaccines have shown promise, with vaccine administration initiating an immune response in vaccinated individuals. Success with BC vaccines have been limited to DCIS and early stage disease. This may be due DCs' failure to generate a robust immune response in advanced disease and to counteract the highly immunosuppressive tumor microenvironment.[96,97]

In a 2007 study, Czerniecki and colleagues,[98] in a HER2 + DCIS presurgical population, demonstrated an 18% pathological complete response (pCR) rate after 4 doses of DC vaccination. In participants with residual DCIS, 50% had no remaining HER2 expression in residual DCIS. The same research group, years later, demonstrated that a type I polarized DC vaccine loaded with HER2 peptides (HER2-DC1) elicited robust anti-HER2 CD4 + T cell immune responses in vaccinated patients with either ER+ or ER-/HER2 + BC. This led to enhanced pCR rates in patients with HER2 + DCIS and early-stage BC. In the same population, DC1 vaccination plus anti-estrogen therapy elicited HER2-specific Th1 immunity. The study demonstrated vaccine safety and a showed a signal of recurrence rate reduction, though it was underpowered for this endpoint.[99–101]

In a more recent trial (NCT02636582), NeuVax, an HER2-derived MHC class I peptide E75 vaccine (nelipepimut-S [NPS]) was combined with granulocyte-macrophage colony-stimulating factor (GM-CSF) and compared with GM-CSF alone in patients with DCIS. In this study, HER2-positivity was not required for eligibility. After randomizing 13 patients 2:1, the investigators showed numerically greater increase—though not statistically significant—NPS-specific cytotoxic T lymphocyte responses in the NPS + GM-CSF arm.[102]

In the HER2-negative setting, the NCT06218303 trial employs the prototype DAA/TAA vaccine targeting MUC1 in postmenopausal women with ER-positive DCIS. Patients are randomized to receive neoadjuvant endocrine therapy for 12 weeks before surgery, alone or in combination with the experimental vaccine. The trial will measure immunogenicity by evaluating the increase of serum anti-MUC1 IgG from baseline. And in BRCA1/2 mutation carriers in the primary prevention setting, another study will evaluate a combination of hTERT, WT1, and prostate-specific membrane antigen with or without IL-12 plasmid (NCT04367675).

Preliminary DCIS vaccine studies appear safe, and can elicit sustained response, though further research is necessary to determine their clinical effectiveness. Most strategies for reducing treatment intensity rely on precise risk assessment, which is increasingly influenced by research in genetics and biomarkers. As our comprehension of the genetic and biological basis of DCIS advances, ongoing research efforts hold promise for personalized management approaches tailored to individual patient risks, where cure optimization will result in better patient outcomes.

ACKNOWLEDGMENT

The authors would like to acknowledge Kaitlyn T. Bifolck, BA, for her editorial support. She is a full-time employee of Dana-Farber Cancer Institute and was not compensated beyond her regular salary.

REFERENCES

1. Spira A, Yurgelun MB, Alexandrov L, et al. Precancer atlas to drive precision prevention trials. Cancer Res 2017;77(7):1510–41.

2. Stanton SE, Castle PE, Finn OJ, et al. Advances and challenges in cancer immunoprevention and immune interception. J Immunother Cancer 2024;12(3). https://doi.org/10.1136/jitc-2023-007815.

3. Sanati S. Morphologic and molecular features of breast ductal carcinoma in situ. Am J Pathol 2019;189(5):946–55.

4. Allred DC, Anderson SJ, Paik S, et al. Adjuvant tamoxifen reduces subsequent breast cancer in women with estrogen receptor-positive ductal carcinoma in situ: a study based on NSABP protocol B-24. J Clin Oncol 2012;30(12):1268–73.

5. Fisher B, Costantino JP, Wickerham DL, et al. Tamoxifen for the prevention of breast cancer: current status of the National Surgical Adjuvant Breast and Bowel Project P-1 study. J Natl Cancer Inst 2005;97(22):1652–62.

6. Cuzick J, Sestak I, Cawthorn S, et al. Tamoxifen for prevention of breast cancer: extended long-term follow-up of the IBIS-I breast cancer prevention trial. Lancet Oncol 2015;16(1):67–75.

7. Powles TJ, Ashley S, Tidy A, et al. Twenty-year follow-up of the Royal Marsden randomized, double-blinded tamoxifen breast cancer prevention trial. J Natl Cancer Inst 2007;99(4):283–90.

8. Veronesi U, Maisonneuve P, Rotmensz N, et al. Italian randomized trial among women with hysterectomy: tamoxifen and hormone-dependent breast cancer in high-risk women. J Natl Cancer Inst 2003;95(2):160–5.

9. DeCensi A, Puntoni M, Guerrieri-Gonzaga A, et al. Randomized Placebo Controlled Trial of Low-Dose Tamoxifen to Prevent Local and Contralateral Recurrence in Breast Intraepithelial Neoplasia. J Clin Oncol 2019;37(19):1629–37.

10. Lazzeroni M, Puntoni M, Guerrieri-Gonzaga A, et al. Randomized placebo controlled trial of low-dose tamoxifen to prevent recurrence in breast noninvasive neoplasia: A 10-Year Follow-Up of TAM-01 study. J Clin Oncol 2023;41(17):3116–21.

11. Allred DC, Brown P, Medina D. The origins of estrogen receptor alpha-positive and estrogen receptor alpha-negative human breast cancer. Breast Cancer Res 2004;6(6):240–5.

12. Sundara Rajan S, Verma R, Shaaban AM, et al. Palpable ductal carcinoma in situ: analysis of radiological and histological features of a large series with 5-year follow-up. Clin Breast Cancer 2013;13(6):486–91.

13. Schwartz GF, Patchefsky AS, Finklestein SD, et al. Nonpalpable in situ ductal carcinoma of the breast. Predictors of multicentricity and microinvasion and implications for treatment. Arch Surg 1989;124(1):29–32.

14. Silverstein MJ, Waisman JR, Gamagami P, et al. Intraductal carcinoma of the breast (208 cases). Clinical factors influencing treatment choice. Cancer 1990;66(1):102–8.

15. Fisher ER, Dignam J, Tan-Chiu E, et al. Pathologic findings from the National Surgical Adjuvant Breast Project (NSABP) eight-year update of Protocol B-17: intraductal carcinoma. Cancer 1999;86(3):429–38.

16. Toss MS, Miligy I, Al-Kawaz A, et al. Prognostic significance of tumor-infiltrating lymphocytes in ductal carcinoma in situ of the breast. Mod Pathol 2018;31(8):1226–36.

17. Risom T, Glass DR, Averbukh I, et al. Transition to invasive breast cancer is associated with progressive changes in the structure and composition of tumor stroma. Cell 2022;185(2):299–310 e18.

18. Lowry KP, Ichikawa L, Hubbard RA, et al. Variation in second breast cancer risk after primary invasive cancer by time since primary cancer diagnosis and estrogen receptor status. Cancer 2023;129(8):1173–82.

19. Wapnir IL, Dignam JJ, Fisher B, et al. Long-term outcomes of invasive ipsilateral breast tumor recurrences after lumpectomy in NSABP B-17 and B-24 randomized clinical trials for DCIS. J Natl Cancer Inst 2011;103(6):478–88.
20. Solin LJ, Gray R, Hughes LL, et al. Surgical excision without radiation for ductal carcinoma in situ of the breast: 12-year results from the ECOG-ACRIN E5194 study. J Clin Oncol 2015;33(33):3938–44.
21. Forbes JF, Sestak I, Howell A, et al. Anastrozole versus tamoxifen for the prevention of locoregional and contralateral breast cancer in postmenopausal women with locally excised ductal carcinoma in situ (IBIS-II DCIS): a double-blind, randomised controlled trial. Lancet 2016;387(10021):866–73.
22. Margolese RG, Cecchini RS, Julian TB, et al. Anastrozole versus tamoxifen in postmenopausal women with ductal carcinoma in situ undergoing lumpectomy plus radiotherapy (NSABP B-35): a randomised, double-blind, phase 3 clinical trial. Lancet 2016;387(10021):849–56.
23. Cuzick J, Chu K, Keevil B, et al. Effect of baseline oestradiol serum concentration on the efficacy of anastrozole for preventing breast cancer in postmenopausal women at high risk: a case-control study of the IBIS-II prevention trial. Lancet Oncol 2023. https://doi.org/10.1016/S1470-2045(23)00578-8.
24. Mitchell JM, DeLeire T, Isaacs C. Adherence to hormonal therapy after surgery among older women with ductal carcinoma in situ: Implications for breast cancer-related adverse health events. Cancer 2024;130(1):107–16.
25. Gail MH, Costantino JP, Bryant J, et al. Weighing the risks and benefits of tamoxifen treatment for preventing breast cancer. J Natl Cancer Inst 1999 Nov 3;91(21):1829–46. Erratum in: J Natl Cancer Inst 2000 Feb 2;92(3):275.
26. Port ER, Montgomery LL, Heerdt AS, et al. Patient reluctance toward tamoxifen use for breast cancer primary prevention. Ann Surg Oncol 2001;8:580–5.
27. DeCensi A, Puntoni M, Johansson H, et al. Effect Modifiers of Low-Dose Tamoxifen in a Randomized Trial in Breast Noninvasive Disease. Clin Cancer Res 2021;27(13):3576–83.
28. Sestak I, Distler W, Forbes JF, et al. Effect of body mass index on recurrences in tamoxifen and anastrozole treated women: an exploratory analysis from the ATAC trial. J Clin Oncol 2010;28(21):3411–5.
29. Pfeiler G, Konigsberg R, Fesl C, et al. Impact of body mass index on the efficacy of endocrine therapy in premenopausal patients with breast cancer: an analysis of the prospective ABCSG-12 trial. J Clin Oncol 2011;29(19):2653–9.
30. Smith SG, Sestak I, Morris MA, et al. The impact of body mass index on breast cancer incidence among women at increased risk: an observational study from the International Breast Intervention Studies. Breast Cancer Res Treat 2021;188(1):215–23.
31. Ethun KF, Wood CE, Register TC, et al. Effects of bazedoxifene acetate with and without conjugated equine estrogens on the breast of postmenopausal monkeys. Menopause 2012;19(11):1242–52.
32. Messier TL, Boyd JR, Gordon JAR, et al. Epigenetic and transcriptome responsiveness to ER modulation by tissue selective estrogen complexes in breast epithelial and breast cancer cells. PLoS One 2022;17(7):e0271725. https://doi.org/10.1371/journal.pone.0271725.
33. Fabian CJ, Nye L, Powers KR, et al. Effect of bazedoxifene and conjugated estrogen (duavee) on breast cancer risk biomarkers in high-risk women: a pilot study. Cancer Prev Res (Phila) 2019;12(10):711–20.
34. Behjati S, Frank MH. The effects of tamoxifen on immunity. Curr Med Chem 2009;16(24):3076–80.

35. Huang H, Zhou J, Chen H, et al. The immunomodulatory effects of endocrine therapy in breast cancer. J Exp Clin Cancer Res 2021;40(1):19.

36. Punglia RS, Bifolck K, Golshan M, et al. Epidemiology, biology, treatment, and prevention of ductal carcinoma in situ (DCIS). JNCI Cancer Spectr 2018;2(4): pky063. https://doi.org/10.1093/jncics/pky063.

37. Fisher B, Dignam J, Wolmark N, et al. Lumpectomy and radiation therapy for the treatment of intraductal breast cancer: findings from National Surgical Adjuvant Breast and Bowel Project B-17. J Clin Oncol 1998;16(2):441–52.

38. Jordan RM, Oxenberg J. Breast cancer conservation therapy. StatPearls Publishing; 2024 Jan. Available at: https://www.ncbi.nlm.nih.gov/books/NBK547708/.

39. Rakovitch E, Pignol JP, Hanna W, et al. Significance of multifocality in ductal carcinoma in situ: outcomes of women treated with breast-conserving therapy. J Clin Oncol 2007;25(35):5591–6.

40. Hwang ES, Malek V. Estimating the magnitude of clinical benefit of local therapy in patients with DCIS. Breast 2019;48(Suppl 1):S34–8.

41. Ward EM, DeSantis CE, Lin CC, et al. Cancer statistics: breast cancer in situ. CA Cancer J Clin Nov-Dec 2015;65(6):481–95.

42. Morrow M, Van Zee KJ, Solin LJ, et al. Society of surgical oncology-american society for radiation oncology-american society of clinical oncology consensus guideline on margins for breast-conserving surgery with whole-breast irradiation in ductal carcinoma in situ. J Clin Oncol 2016;34(33):4040–6.

43. Rudloff U, Jacks LM, Goldberg JI, et al. Nomogram for predicting the risk of local recurrence after breast-conserving surgery for ductal carcinoma in situ. J Clin Oncol 2010;28(23):3762–9.

44. Bremer T, Whitworth PW, Patel R, et al. A biological signature for breast ductal carcinoma in situ to predict radiotherapy benefit and assess recurrence risk. Clin Cancer Res 2018;24(23):5895–901.

45. Miller ME, Kyrillos A, Yao K, et al. Utilization of axillary surgery for patients with ductal carcinoma in situ: a report from the national cancer data base. Ann Surg Oncol 2016;23(10):3337–46.

46. National Comprehensive Cancer Network. Clinical practice guidelines in oncology-breast cancer version 4. 2020. Available at: http://www.nccn.com.

47. El Hage Chehade H, Headon H, Wazir U, et al. Is sentinel lymph node biopsy indicated in patients with a diagnosis of ductal carcinoma in situ? a systematic literature review and meta-analysis. Am J Surg 2017;213(1):171–80.

48. Hung P, Wang SY, Killelea BK, et al. Long-term outcomes of sentinel lymph node biopsy for ductal carcinoma in situ. JNCI Cancer Spectr 2019;3(4):pkz052. https://doi.org/10.1093/jncics/pkz052.

49. Eusebi V, Feudale E, Foschini MP, et al. Long-term follow-up of in situ carcinoma of the breast. Semin Diagn Pathol 1994;11(3):223–35.

50. Sanders ME, Schuyler PA, Dupont WD, et al. The natural history of low-grade ductal carcinoma in situ of the breast in women treated by biopsy only revealed over 30 years of long-term follow-up. Cancer 2005;103(12):2481–4.

51. Sanders ME, Schuyler PA, Simpson JF, et al. Continued observation of the natural history of low-grade ductal carcinoma in situ reaffirms proclivity for local recurrence even after more than 30 years of follow-up. Mod Pathol 2015;28(5):662–9.

52. Francis A, Thomas J, Fallowfield L, et al. Addressing overtreatment of screen detected DCIS; the LORIS trial. Eur J Cancer 2015;51(16):2296–303.

53. Hwang ES, Hyslop T, Lynch T, et al. The COMET (Comparison of Operative versus Monitoring and Endocrine Therapy) trial: a phase III randomised controlled clinical

trial for low-risk ductal carcinoma in situ (DCIS). BMJ Open 2019;9(3):e026797. https://doi.org/10.1136/bmjopen-2018-026797.

54. Elshof LE, Tryfonidis K, Slaets L, et al. Feasibility of a prospective, randomised, open-label, international multicentre, phase III, non-inferiority trial to assess the safety of active surveillance for low risk ductal carcinoma in situ - The LORD study. Eur J Cancer 2015;51(12):1497–510.

55. Kanbayashi C, Iwata H. Current approach and future perspective for ductal carcinoma in situ of the breast. Jpn J Clin Oncol 2017;47(8):671–7.

56. Early Breast Cancer Trialists' Collaborative Group, Correa C, McGale P, Wang Y, et al. Overview of the randomized trials of radiotherapy in ductal carcinoma in situ of the breast. J Natl Cancer Inst Monogr 2010;2010(41):162–77.

57. McCormick B, Winter K, Hudis C, et al. RTOG 9804: a prospective randomized trial for good-risk ductal carcinoma in situ comparing radiotherapy with observation. J Clin Oncol 2015;33(7):709–15.

58. McCormick B, Winter KA, Woodward W, et al. Randomized phase III trial evaluating radiation following surgical excision for good-risk ductal carcinoma in situ: long-term report from NRG oncology/RTOG 9804. J Clin Oncol 2021;39(32):3574–82.

59. Rakovitch E, Nofech-Mozes S, Hanna W, et al. A population-based validation study of the DCIS Score predicting recurrence risk in individuals treated by breast-conserving surgery alone. Breast Cancer Res Treat 2015;152(2):389–98.

60. Rakovitch E, Nofech-Mozes S, Hanna W, et al. Multigene expression assay and benefit of radiotherapy after breast conservation in ductal carcinoma in situ. J Natl Cancer Inst 2017;109(4). https://doi.org/10.1093/jnci/djw256.

61. Solin LJ, Gray R, Baehner FL, et al. A multigene expression assay to predict local recurrence risk for ductal carcinoma in situ of the breast. J Natl Cancer Inst 2013;105(10):701–10.

62. Rakovitch E, Parpia S, Koch A, et al. DUCHESS: an evaluation of the ductal carcinoma in situ score for decisions on radiotherapy in patients with low/intermediate-risk DCIS. Breast Cancer Res Treat 2021;188(1):133–9.

63. Shah C, Bremer T, Cox C, et al. The clinical utility of DCISionRT((R)) on radiation therapy decision making in patients with ductal carcinoma in situ following breast-conserving surgery. Ann Surg Oncol 2021;28(11):5974–84.

64. Raldow AC, Sher D, Chen AB, et al. Cost effectiveness of the oncotype DX DCIS score for guiding treatment of patients with ductal carcinoma in situ. J Clin Oncol 2016;34(33):3963–8.

65. D'Rummo KA, Miller L, TenNapel MJ, et al. Assessing the financial toxicity of radiation oncology patients using the validated comprehensive score for financial toxicity as a patient-reported outcome. Pract Radiat Oncol Sep-Oct 2020;10(5):e322–9.

66. Liu MC. Transforming the landscape of early cancer detection using blood tests-Commentary on current methodologies and future prospects. Br J Cancer 2021;124(9):1475–7.

67. Beer TM. Novel blood-based early cancer detection: diagnostics in development. Am J Manag Care 2020;26(14 Suppl):S292–9.

68. Liu MC, Oxnard GR, Klein EA, et al. Sensitive and specific multi-cancer detection and localization using methylation signatures in cell-free DNA. Ann Oncol 2020;31(6):745–59.

69. Cristiano S, Leal A, Phallen J, et al. Genome-wide cell-free DNA fragmentation in patients with cancer. Nature 2019;570(7761):385–9.

70. Lennon AM, Buchanan AH, Kinde I, et al. Feasibility of blood testing combined with PET-CT to screen for cancer and guide intervention. Science 2020; 369(6499). https://doi.org/10.1126/science.abb9601.

71. Rossi SH, Stewart GD. Re: clinical validation of a targeted methylation-based multi-cancer early detection test using an independent validation Set. Eur Urol 2022;82(4):442–3.

72. Hackshaw A, Clarke CA, Hartman AR. New genomic technologies for multi-cancer early detection: Rethinking the scope of cancer screening. Cancer Cell 2022;40(2):109–13.

73. Chin YM, Takahashi Y, Chan HT, et al. Ultradeep targeted sequencing of circulating tumor DNA in plasma of early and advanced breast cancer. Cancer Sci 2021;112(1):454–64.

74. Schrag D, Beer TM, McDonnell CH 3rd, et al. Blood-based tests for multicancer early detection (PATHFINDER): a prospective cohort study. Lancet 2023; 402(10409):1251–60.

75. Neal RD, Johnson P, Clarke CA, et al. Cell-Free DNA-based multi-cancer early detection test in an asymptomatic screening population (NHS-Galleri): design of a pragmatic, prospective randomised controlled trial. Cancers (Basel) 2022; 14(19). https://doi.org/10.3390/cancers14194818.

76. Nicholson BD, Oke J, Virdee PS, et al. Multi-cancer early detection test in symptomatic patients referred for cancer investigation in England and Wales (SYMPLIFY): a large-scale, observational cohort study. Lancet Oncol 2023;24(7): 733–43.

77. Shimomura A, Shiino S, Kawauchi J, et al. Novel combination of serum microRNA for detecting breast cancer in the early stage. Cancer Sci 2016;107(3): 326–34.

78. Clift AK, Dodwell D, Lord S, et al. The current status of risk-stratified breast screening. Br J Cancer 2022;126(4):533–50.

79. Aleshin-Guendel S, Lange J, Goodman P, et al. A Latent Disease Model to Reduce Detection Bias in Cancer Risk Prediction Studies. Eval Health Prof 2021; 44(1):42–9.

80. Trentham-Dietz A, Alagoz O, Chapman C, et al. Reflecting on 20 years of breast cancer modeling in CISNET: Recommendations for future cancer systems modeling efforts. PLoS Comput Biol 2021;17(6):e1009020. https://doi.org/10.1371/journal.pcbi.1009020.

81. Shen Y, Dong W, Gulati R, et al. Estimating the frequency of indolent breast cancer in screening trials. Stat Methods Med Res 2019;28(4):1261–71.

82. Fitzgerald RC, Antoniou AC, Fruk L, et al. The future of early cancer detection. Nat Med 2022;28(4):666–77.

83. Petridis C, Brook MN, Shah V, et al. Genetic predisposition to ductal carcinoma in situ of the breast. Breast Cancer Res 2016;18(1):22.

84. Lamb LR, Lehman CD, Oseni TO, et al. Ductal Carcinoma In Situ (DCIS) at Breast MRI: Predictors of Upgrade to Invasive Carcinoma. Acad Radiol 2020; 27(10):1394–9.

85. Chou SS, Gombos EC, Chikarmane SA, et al. Computer-aided heterogeneity analysis in breast MR imaging assessment of ductal carcinoma in situ: Correlating histologic grade and receptor status. J Magn Reson Imaging 2017; 46(6):1748–59.

86. Rahbar H, Partridge SC, Demartini WB, et al. In vivo assessment of ductal carcinoma in situ grade: a model incorporating dynamic contrast-enhanced and

diffusion-weighted breast MR imaging parameters. Radiology 2012;263(2):374–82.
87. Grimm LJ, Rahbar H, Abdelmalak M, et al. Ductal Carcinoma in Situ: State-of-the-Art Review. Radiology 2022;302(2):246–55.
88. Yang ML, Bhimani C, Roth R, et al. Contrast enhanced mammography: focus on frequently encountered benign and malignant diagnoses. Cancer Imag 2023;23(1):10.
89. Cozzi A, Magni V, Zanardo M, et al. Contrast-enhanced Mammography: A Systematic Review and Meta-Analysis of Diagnostic Performance. Radiology 2022;302(3):568–81.
90. Vignoli C, Bicchierai G, De Benedetto D, et al. Role of preoperative breast dual-energy contrast-enhanced digital mammography in ductal carcinoma in situ. Breast J 2019;25(5):1034–6.
91. Cheung YC, Juan YH, Lin YC, et al. Dual-Energy Contrast-Enhanced Spectral Mammography: Enhancement Analysis on BI-RADS 4 Non-Mass Microcalcifications in Screened Women. PLoS One 2016;11(9):e0162740.
92. Erbas B, Provenzano E, Armes J, et al. The natural history of ductal carcinoma in situ of the breast: a review. Breast Cancer Res Treat 2006;97(2):135–44.
93. Ozanne EM, Shieh Y, Barnes J, et al. Characterizing the impact of 25 years of DCIS treatment. Breast Cancer Res Treat 2011;129(1):165–73.
94. Wallis MG, Clements K, Kearins O, et al. The effect of DCIS grade on rate, type and time to recurrence after 15 years of follow-up of screen-detected DCIS. Br J Cancer 2012;106(10):1611–7.
95. National Comprehensive Cancer Network. NCCN Guidelines for Patients® Ductal Carcinoma in Situ Breast Cancer. 2024. Available at: https://www.nccn.org/patientresources/patient-resources/guidelines-for-patients/guidelines-for-patients-details?patientGuidelineId=30.
96. Zachariah NN, Basu A, Gautam N, et al. Intercepting premalignant, preinvasive breast lesions through vaccination. Front Immunol 2021;12:786286.
97. De La Cruz LM, Nocera NF, Czerniecki BJ. Restoring anti-oncodriver Th1 responses with dendritic cell vaccines in HER2/neu-positive breast cancer: progress and potential. Immunotherapy 2016;8(10):1219–32.
98. Czerniecki BJ, Koski GK, Koldovsky U, et al. Targeting HER-2/neu in early breast cancer development using dendritic cells with staged interleukin-12 burst secretion. Cancer Res 2007;67(4):1842–52.
99. Sharma A, Koldovsky U, Xu S, et al. HER-2 pulsed dendritic cell vaccine can eliminate HER-2 expression and impact ductal carcinoma in situ. Cancer 2012;118(17):4354–62.
100. Datta J, Berk E, Xu S, et al. Anti-HER2 CD4(+) T-helper type 1 response is a novel immune correlate to pathologic response following neoadjuvant therapy in HER2-positive breast cancer. Breast Cancer Res 2015;17(1):71.
101. Lowenfeld L, Zaheer S, Oechsle C, et al. Addition of anti-estrogen therapy to anti-HER2 dendritic cell vaccination improves regional nodal immune response and pathologic complete response rate in patients with ER(pos)/HER2(pos) early breast cancer. OncoImmunology 2017;6(9):e1207032.
102. O'Shea AE, Clifton GT, Qiao N, et al. Phase II Trial of Nelipepimut-S Peptide Vaccine in Women with Ductal Carcinoma In Situ. Cancer Prev Res (Phila) 2023;16(6):333–41.

Skin Cancer Precursors
From Cancer Genomics to Early Diagnosis

Madison M. Taylor, BSA[a,b], Kelly C. Nelson, MD[b,*],
Florentia Dimitriou, MD, PhD[c,d]

KEYWORDS

- Initiation • Progression • Melanoma • Cutaneous squamous cell carcinoma
- Basal cell carcinoma • Solid organ transplant recipients

KEY POINTS

- Skin cancer initiation and progression are multifactorial and are influenced by host and environmental factors.
- Melanoma progression trajectories vary mainly depending on their relation to ultraviolet exposure.
- Actinic keratoses (AKs) serve as strong predictors of eventual cutaneous squamous cell carcinoma (cSCC) development and may rarely progress to cSCC.
- Targeted deep sequencing analysis revealed a model to explain the progression from AK to cSCC.
- Patients with immune dysregulation carry an increased risk of cutaneous malignancies.

INTRODUCTION

Skin cancers, including melanoma and keratinocyte carcinomas (KCs) (basal cell carcinomas [BCC] and squamous cell carcinomas), are responsible for increasing health care burden internationally. Genomic sequencing and molecular profiling have illustrated the complexity of genomic, transcriptomic, and epigenetic events that correlate with skin cancer development. Cancer initiation is characterized by an abnormal cell behavior and is followed by the subsequent emergence of additional alterations that drive cancer progression. During this multistage cancer development, genetic alterations that occur at several levels, such as single nucleotides or whole genes, lead

[a] John P. and Kathrine G. McGovern Medical School, The University of Texas Health Science Center, 6431 Fannin Street, Houston, TX 77030, USA; [b] Department of Dermatology, The University of Texas MD Anderson Cancer Center, 1400 Pressler Street, Unit 1452, Houston, TX 77030, USA; [c] Department of Surgical Oncology, The University of Texas MD Anderson Cancer Center, 1400 Pressler Street, Unit 1484, Houston, TX 77030, USA; [d] Department of Dermatology, University Hospital of Zurich, University of Zurich, Rämistrasse 100, 8091 Zürich, Switzerland
* Corresponding author. Department of Dermatology, The University of Texas MD Anderson Cancer Center, 1400 Pressler Street, Unit 1452, Houston, TX 77030.
E-mail address: KCNelson1@mdanderson.org

Hematol Oncol Clin N Am 38 (2024) 851–868
https://doi.org/10.1016/j.hoc.2024.04.005
0889-8588/24/© 2024 Elsevier Inc. All rights reserved.

to genomic instability and generation of distinct subclones that drive tumor growth and progression. A comprehensive understanding of the sequence of molecular alterations in the cells that lead to skin cancer initiation, invasiveness, and progression is fundamental to improve early detection and prevention (**Fig. 1**). Furthermore, the ability to distinguish which lesions might regress or obtain a state of equilibrium is essential to prevent unnecessary treatment. In this review, the authors summarize the clinical and genetic characteristics of skin cancer precursors in melanoma and KCs, as well as future directions for risk assessment and early detection.

THE MAIN CONCEPTS OF SKIN CANCER INITIATION

The role of the *exposome*—the accumulation of environmental influences alongside associated biological responses—has been increasingly recognized as a contributor to cancer initiation (**Fig. 2**). Its contribution is especially evident in the cause-effect relationship of ultraviolet (UV) radiation (UVR)–induced mutagenesis. UVR induces dimerization of adjacent DNA pyrimidine residues and subsequent conversion of TT to CC. These mutation signatures are found in several tumor suppressor genes and oncogenes in cutaneous cancers, including the *p53* gene.[1] Interestingly, these activating mutations are present even in early, benign stages such as the sun-exposed skin of aging individuals. Similarly, *ras* gene mutations can be found in benign papillomas, even though genetic mutations causing RAS pathway hyperactivation drive oncogenic transformation and sustain cancer growth in melanomas and are present in almost 100% of melanoma cases.[2–4] The presence of *p53* and *ras* mutations in benign tissues indicates that oncogenic mutations may be insufficient to promote cancer alone. Thus, prior to our review of skin cancer precursors and progression, it's paramount to discuss other components of cancerogenesis, including genomic instability, tumor microenvironment (TME), microbiome, and mechanisms underlying metastasis.

Genomic instability is caused either by inherited mutations in genes that monitor genomic integrity, or by acquired somatic mutations during tumor development.

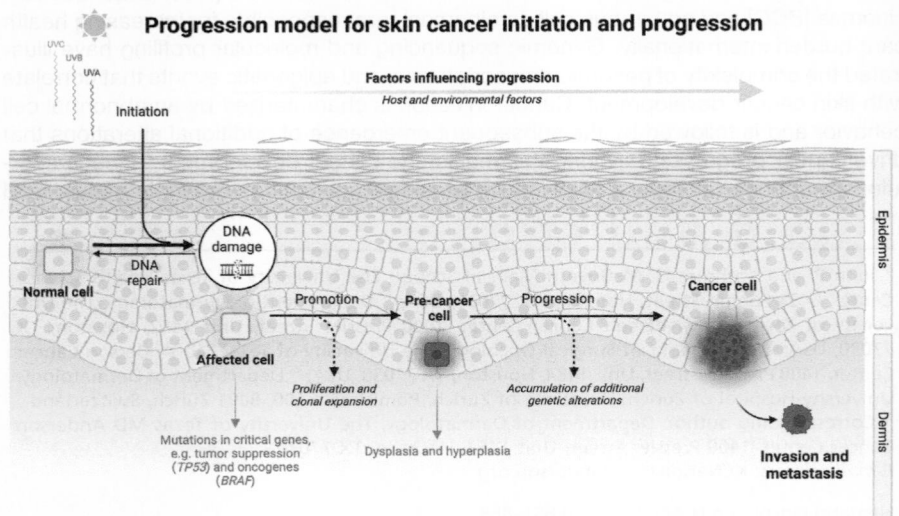

Fig. 1. A general model for skin cancer initiation and progression.

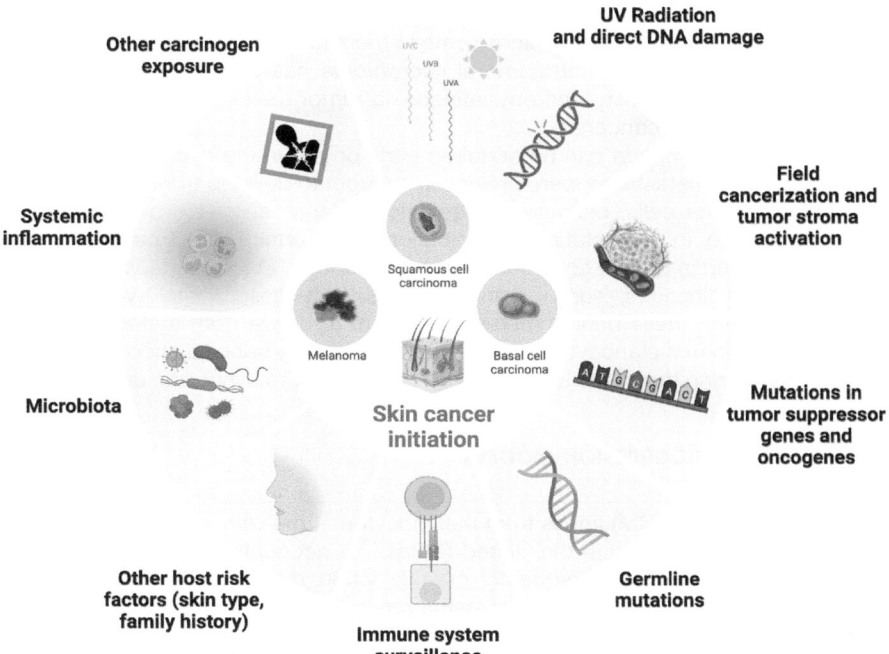

Fig. 2. Host intrinsic and extrinsic factors contributing to skin cancer initiation.

These genetic changes can occur at several levels, giving rise to nucleotide, microsatellite, or chromosome instability.[5,6] A clinical example of genomic stability is xeroderma pigmentosum (XP), a rare autosomal recessive disorder where ineffective nucleotide excision repair results in numerous cutaneous malignancies.[7]

TME—defined as interactive populations of cancer and stromal cells—has an integral role in tumorigenesis and malignant progression.[8] While cancer-associated fibroblasts, innate immune cells, and endothelial cells are epigenetically programmed upon their recruitment by soluble factors,[8,9] the exact mechanism that allows these normal cells to support tumor development and progression is not yet fully understood. Similar non-mutational epigenetic changes can also result in clonal outgrowth of cancer cells and enable their proliferative expansion and invasive growth capability. For example, a hypoxic TME, due to insufficient vascularization, is linked to tumor progression and poor clinical outcomes in advanced melanoma patients.[10]

Lately, there is growing evidence that the gut and intratumoral *microbiome*—resident bacteria and fungi that symbiotically exist with bodily tissues—have profound impact on health and disease.[11] Specific gut microorganisms can correlate with cancer development, disease progression, and response to anticancer treatment.[8,12] Interestingly, many immune checkpoint blockade (ICB) response–associated bacteria among metastatic melanoma patients have known roles in starch degradation and fiber fermentation; and among metastatic melanoma patients receiving ICB treatment, patients with the highest fiber intake demonstrate significantly higher progression-free survival when compared to patients with the lowest fiber intake.[13] While early-stage melanoma patients demonstrate different gut microbiome diversity than those with late-stage melanoma, and patients with no history of melanoma demonstrated different gut microbial diversity than those with any history of melanoma, the specific role of the gut microbiome to melanoma development is still being explored.[14] Additionally, the intratumoral *microbiome* has been increasingly implicated in tumor susceptibility, thereby influencing tumor development and progression in various human cancers.[15]

Metastatic Dissemination can be acquired early or late in the evolution of primary neoplasms. While metastases were previously thought to develop from clonal expansion of single tumor cells, biologic and genetic evidence suggests polyclonal processes contribute to metastatic dissemination.[16,17] Furthermore, metastasis has also been reported in benign conditions, such as eruptive Spitz nevi, thus underlining that certain cell lineages, such as melanocytes, can disseminate even at early stages.[18] However, these benign metastases seem to derive from a clonal origin of partially transformed melanocytes and are characterized by specific oncogenic mutations, reemphasizing the association of specific mutations to dysplastic development.

PRECURSOR AND PROGRESSION MODELS
Melanoma

Cutaneous melanoma (CM) arises from melanocytes of the skin and is the fifth most common cancer diagnosed in the United States.[19] It accounts for over 80% of skin cancer deaths but remains frequently curable when diagnosed at early disease stages.[20] Cutaneous melanocytic neoplasms range from benign nevi to invasive tumors (melanomas), with dysplastic nevi (DN) being recognized as intermediate neoplasms (**Fig. 3**). Despite this intermediate recognition, melanomas most commonly arise de novo from clinically normal skin without requiring a dysplastic nevus: normal skin may have melanocytes with pathogenic mutations sufficient to support melanoma development.[21] Moreover, melanocytes from intermittently sun-exposed skin have a lower mutational burden than melanocytes from CSD skin.[22] Understanding the processes that lead premalignant melanocytes of normal skin to enter early stages of malignant transformation is essential to understand the causes and origins of melanoma.

CM represents a clinically, molecularly, and histopathologically heterogenous group of tumors. CM is classified histopathologically as superficial spreading, nodular, lentigo maligna (LM), or acral lentiginous subtypes. However, the authors will organize the narrative based on shared premalignancy trajectories: CM arising on non-chronically sun damaged (CSD) skin, CM arising on CSD skin, nodular melanoma (NM), and DN (**Fig. 4**).[23]

Melanoma arising on non-chronically sun-damaged skin
CM of non-CSD skin typically arise de novo, with 26% developing from an existing nevus,[24] forming melanoma in situ *(MIS) with pagetoid features*, then progressing to

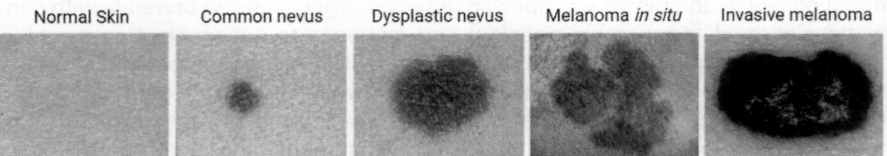

Normal Skin   Common nevus   Dysplastic nevus   Melanoma *in situ*   Invasive melanoma

Fig. 3. Lesions on the melanocytic spectrum. (*Adapted from* Shain, A.H. and B.C. Bastian, From melanocytes to melanomas. Nature reviews. Cancer, 2016. 16(6): p. 345-358, 10.1038/nrc.2016.37; with permission. [Figure 2 in original].)

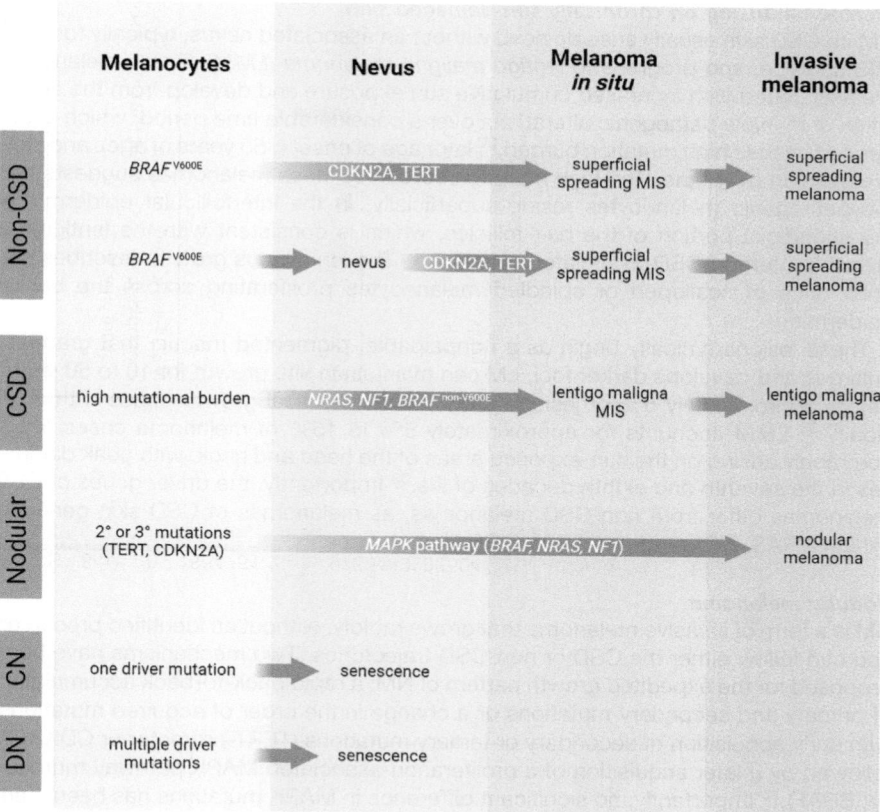

Fig. 4. Common melanoma progression trajectories. A visualization from cells of origin to precursors and distinct melanoma subtypes, including sequential genetic observations. Although these are the most common trajectories, it's important to note melanoma can arise following other pathways, including within CN and DN. CSD, chronically sun damaged skin. CN, common nevus; DN, dysplastic nevus; MIS, melanoma in situ.

superficial spreading melanoma (SSM). Non-CSD melanomas begin with a pagetoid growth pattern: enlarged and rounded melanocytes spread throughout the layers of the epidermis, arranged partially in nests. The earliest stage of MIS with pagetoid features appears clinically as an asymmetric macule or patch with variable pigmentation, including shades of red, blue, black, gray, or white. As indicated by 'superficial spreading,' the MIS first grows horizontally, ranging in diameter from millimeters to centimeters, for months to years before subsequent invasion through the dermis.

SSM typically occurs earlier in life (<55 years of age) and accounts for approximately 70% of all melanomas, with 30% of SSM maintaining an area representative of a pre-existing common nevus.[23,24] The $BRAF^{V600E}$ somatic mutation is associated with benign nevi, pagetoid growth pattern, and non-CSD melanomas.[25] While a $BRAF^{V600E}$ mutation is sufficient to form a nevus,[26,27] individual nevi rarely progress to melanoma.[28] Thus, nevi with BRAF mutations require secondary or tertiary alterations to progress to melanoma, commonly mutations in *CDKN2A* or the *TERT* promoter sequence.[29]

Melanoma arising on chronically sun-damaged skin

CM on CSD skin usually arise de novo without an associated nevus, typically form LM MIS subtype, and progress to lentigo maligna melanoma (LMM). These melanomas are associated with increased cumulative sun exposure and develop from the acquisition of multiple pathogenic alterations over a considerable time period, which is evidenced by their high mutation burden,[30] later age of onset (>55 years of age), and slow progression over time. The high mutation burden of these melanomas suggests that the pathogenic melanocytes reside superficially, in the interfollicular epidermis or the superficial portion of the hair follicles, which is consistent with the lentiginous growth pattern of CSD-associated melanoma. The lentiginous growth describes singular units of scalloped or spindled melanocytes proliferating across the basilar epidermis.

These lesions typically begin as a nonpalpable, pigmented macule that gradually enlarges and develops darker foci. LM can maintain in situ growth for 10 to 50 years, before approximately 5% of lesions progress to a vertical growth phase with invasion.[31,32] LMM accounts for approximately 5% to 15% of melanoma cases, most commonly arising on the sun-exposed areas of the head and neck, with peak diagnoses in the seventh and eighth decades of life.[33] Importantly, the driver genes of CSD melanomas differ from non-CSD melanomas, as melanomas of CSD skin generally exhibit NRAS, NF1, and non-V600 E BRAF mutations.[22]

Nodular melanoma

NM is a form of invasive melanoma that grows rapidly, without an identified precursor, and can follow either the CSD or non-CSD trajectories. Two mechanisms have been proposed for the expedited growth pattern of NM: a rapid back-to-back accumulation of primary and secondary mutations or a change in the order of acquired mutations, with early acquisition of secondary or tertiary mutations (TERT promoter or CDKN2A) followed by a later acquisition of a proliferation-associated MAPK pathway mutation (ie, BRAF).[23] Importantly, no significant difference in MAPK mutations has been identified for NM compared to other CM types,[34] indicating the rapidly proliferative growth pattern of NM does not differ due to a novel mutation, but more likely due to a circumstantial progression. NM is the second most common CM subtype, accounting for 15% to 30% of cases, and is well known for its ability to become invasive shortly after arising. By definition, NM is in vertical growth phase, presenting as a papule or nodule, usually with dark pigmentation, commonly arising on the trunk or legs, and is more common in men than in women.

Dysplastic nevi

DN occupy a unique place in the melanocytic tumor spectrum: a small subset of DN may progress to melanoma, but most remain benign, or eventually regress clinically as patients age. Importantly, two-thirds of CM arise de novo, in the absence of a precursor lesion, and the annual risk of any individual nevus progression is less than 0.0005.[28,35] Benign typical nevi invariably have one driver mutation, such as BRAF^{V600E}, while DN have multiple mutations.[29] The mutations found in DN often include proto-oncogenes that activate the MAPK pathway, resulting in melanocyte cell division. DN then enter a phase of oncogene-induced senescence,[36] mediated by 2 tumor suppressors, p53 and pRB. The loss of cell cycle checkpoint genes, such as TP53 and CDKN2A, can bypass this cell cycle arrest.[29,37,38] Telomerase reverse transcriptase (TERT) promoter mutations are more prevalent in DN from older patients, whereas DN with BRAF^{V600E} mutations are observed in younger individuals and show different clinical features than DN with other driver mutations.[38] Overall, DN are important clinical findings, as patients with DN have an increased risk of developing melanoma in their lifetime, with increasing number of DN corresponding with increasing risk.[39,40]

Keratinocyte Carcinomas

The term KC encompasses BCC and cutaneous squamous cell carcinoma (cSCC), which are neoplasms derived from hair follicles of the basal epidermal layer and epidermal keratinocytes, respectively. These are profoundly the most diagnosed cancers each year, totaling more cases than all other cancers combined. However, their exact incidence is difficult to ascertain, as KCs are excluded from most cancer registries. The most recent study of KC incidence in the United States estimates that there were approximately 5.4 million cases in 2012, with a consistent increasing trend.[41] While highly curable, KCs cost an average of 10 years of potential life lost and convey significant morbidity.[42] Thus, early detection and treatment are important for improving patient outcomes and disease morbidity.

Squamous cell carcinoma

cSCC accounts for 20% to 30% of all KCs and is estimated to cause up to 9000 deaths in the United States annually.[43] Cumulative sun exposure is the most significant environmental factor promoting cSCC pathogenesis, as evidenced by UVR-associated mutations and increased incidence with age. Exome sequencing data demonstrate *TP53* mutations and loss-of-function *CDKN2A* mutations in cSCC,[44] as well as higher tumor mutational burden than other solid tumors.[45] Along the spectrum of UVR-induced keratinocyte neoplasms, benign actinic keratoses (AKs) are the most common lesions, with an incidence rate among Medicare patients of 28.7% in 10 years.[46] Furthermore, while most cSCC arise de novo, the presence of AKs is the strongest predictive factor of cSCC development.[47] While 2% to 3% of AKs progress to cSCC within 4 years,[48,49] the exact mechanism underlying the progression of AKs to cSCC remains unclear. Targeted deep sequencing analysis of cSCC lesions paired with adjacent AKs, sun-damaged epidermis, and cSCC in situ indicate that precancerous lesions harbor ≥ 1 driver mutations, but lower copy number alterations than cSCC and specific acquired mutations, such as *NOTCH1* or *TP53*, can promote tumor progression.[1]

In clinical practice, the use of a dermatoscope—a device which visually magnifies lesions and transilluminates features with polarized light—improves diagnostic accuracy for skin cancer and can reveal features along the cSCC progression spectrum. AKs that progress to cSCCs often include vessels that form around follicles, creating a dotted appearance.[50] AKs may progress into an intraepidermal carcinoma (IEC), also known as Bowen's disease, or SCC in situ. IEC presents as a slow-growing, erythematous lesion, with discrete yellow-white scales and dotted vessels.[51] In contrast, an *invasive cSCC* presents as a fast-growing, often tender, papule or nodule with a central yellow/white keratin mass, pinpoints of ulceration, and peripheral looped vessels on dermoscopic examination (**Fig. 5**).

Basal cell carcinoma

BCC arises from the epidermal basal layer interfollicular cells. The American Cancer Society estimates that BCC compromised 80% of 2012 KC cases, or 4.32 million BCC diagnoses.[41] UVR-induced DNA damage prompts alterations of the sonic hedgehog pathways in up to 80% to 90% of cases, including the PTCH1 receptor, SMO signal transducer, and GLI transcription factors.[52–54] Although BCCs arise de novo without identifiable precursors, early diagnosis can reduce morbidity from locally destructive spread.

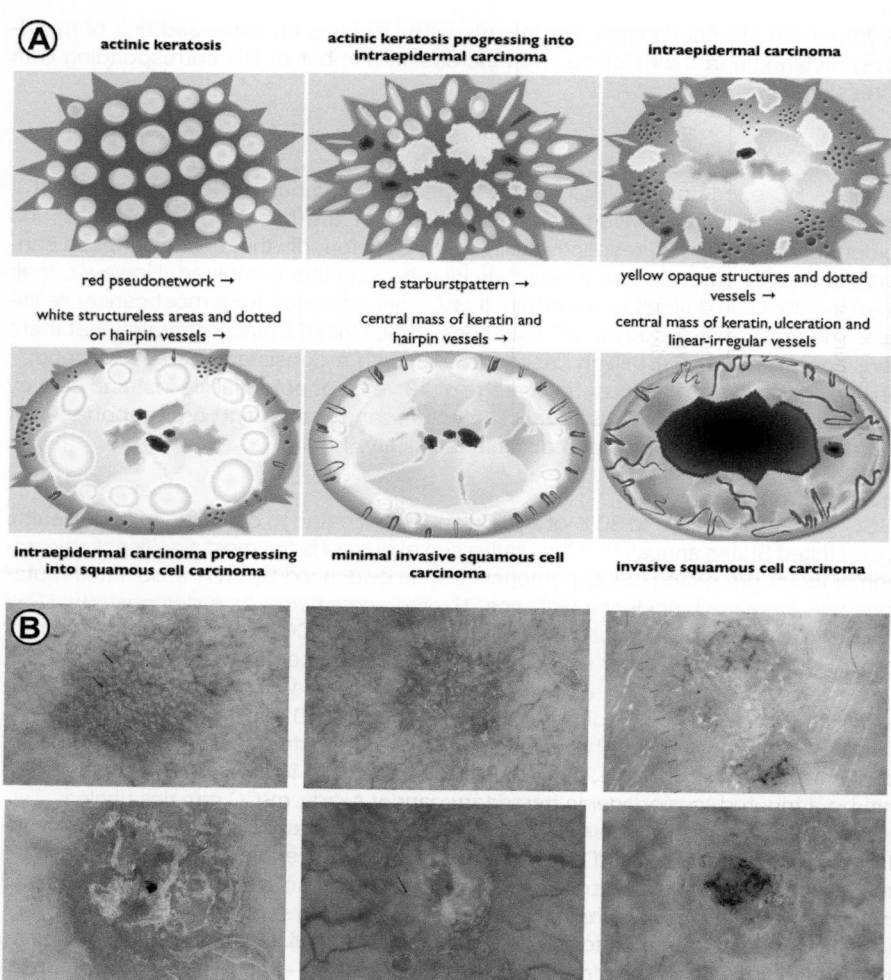

Fig. 5. (*A*) Dermoscopic progression model from actinic keratosis (AK), to intraepidermal carcinoma (IEC), to invasive cutaneous squamous cell carcinoma (cSCC). (*B*) Respective clinical images. (*Adapted from* [*A*] Zalaudek, I.M.D., et al., Dermatoscopy of facial actinic keratosis, intraepidermal carcinoma, and invasive squamous cell carcinoma: A progression model. Journal of the American Academy of Dermatology, 2012. 66(4): p. 589-597; with permission. (Figures 1-7 in original) [*B*] Dermoscopedia. Available at: https://dermoscopedia.org/w/index.php?curid=5341; with permission.)

Most BCCs remain localized, with approximately 70% arising on the face and 15% on the trunk. Clinical and histopathologic presentation can be divided into 3 main categories: nodular, superficial, and infiltrative (**Fig. 6**). Approximately 80% of BCC cases are nodular, presenting as a pink-colored or flesh-colored papule, with a "pearly" or translucent quality, and may have visible telangiectasias. Superficial BCCs constitute 15% of cases and appear as a shiny pink macule or patch. Infiltrative BCC represents 5% to 10% of cases and appears as a pink-to-white, scar-like, indurated papule or plaque, often with atrophic features. These lesions are known for their clinical subtlety and subclinical spread.

| Nodular | Superficial | Infiltrative |

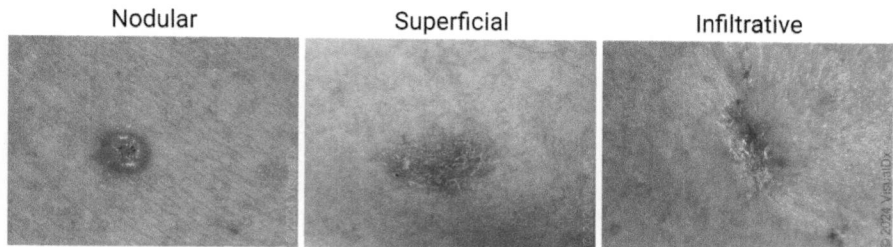

Fig. 6. Common subtypes of basal cell carcinoma. (Used with permission from VisualDx.)

While there are no BCC precursors, germline variants in genes determining pigmentation are associated with increased risk of BCC—such as the melanocortin-1 receptor, human homolog of agouti signaling protein, and tyrosinase—also a gene involved in UV-induced immune tolerance, cytotoxic lymphocyte–associated antigen-4.[55–57] Other polymorphisms are associated with BCC truncal clustering phenotype, including detoxifying genes *CYP450*, *CYP2D6*, glutathione-S-transferase, and tumor necrosis factor.[58,59] Although rare, several cancer-related syndromes are also associated with increased BCC risk and earlier age of onset: nevoid BCC syndrome, Rombo syndrome, Bazex-Dupré-Christol syndrome, XP, Muir-Torre syndrome, and oculocutaneous albinism.

CANCER IMMUNOEDITING AND IMMUNOSUPPRESSION
Cancer Immunoediting

The immune system has 3 important roles in tumor prevention: elimination or suppression of oncogenic viruses, elimination of pathogens and regulation of inflammation, and identification and control of tumor cells.[60] Immunity can also promote tumor progression by shaping tumor immunogenicity. Together, these host-protective and tumor-promoting actions are referred to as cancer immunoediting, a process which occurs in 3 sequential phases: elimination, equilibrium, and escape. Escape from immune control, in which tumors grow and establish an immunosuppressive microenvironment, is being recognized as one of the hallmarks of cancer.[61] The suppression of immune control is central to cancer growth and metastasis, and immunosuppression is an important risk factor for all skin cancers. This concept is well displayed in patients with immune dysregulation—such as solid organ transplant recipients (SOTRs), chronic lymphocytic leukemia patients, and human immunodeficiency virus patients—who carry an increased risk of cutaneous malignancies. Of these cancer-precursing states of immune dysregulation, SOTRs carry the highest risk.

Solid Organ Transplantation

Survival rates have significantly improved for SOTRs.[62] However, the requirement of immunosuppression conveys a 3-fold increased risk of malignancy[63] and increased rates of cancer recurrence, metastasis, and mortality.[62] Of these post-transplant malignancies (PTMs), cutaneous cancers are the most common, accounting for 40% to 50%.[64] Multiple drivers of cutaneous tumorigenesis in SOTRs have been identified, including genetic predisposition, drug-induced alterations, and differences in protein and mRNA expression.

The degree of patient *immunosuppression* is potentially the most significant host factor increasing the risk of PTMs; immunosuppression is highest in the first-year post-transplantation, coinciding with the highest incidence of PTM.[65,66] Although

Table 1
Summary of early skin cancer detection characteristics

Skin Cancer Type	Subtype (%)	Helpful Epidemiology	Common Location	Precursor Lesion	Lesion Description	Course
Melanoma	Superficial spreading (70)	<55 years old	Non-CSD skin	26% develop from an existing nevus	Asymmetric macule or patch with variable pigmentation, including shades of red, blue, black, gray, or white	Begins with slow horizontal growth, ranging from millimeters to centimeters, growing for months to years before invasion
	Lentigo maligna (5–15)	>55 years old	CSD skin of the head and neck	Usually arise de novo without an associated nevus	Nonpalpable, pigmented macule that gradually enlarges and develops darker foci	Can maintain in situ growth for 10–50 years before invasion
	Nodular (15–30)	Median age 53 Men>Women	CSD or non-CSD skin of the legs or trunk	No identified precursor	Papule or nodule, usually with dark pigmentation	Grows rapidly and is well known to become invasive shortly after arising
BCC	Nodular (80)	>55 years old Men>Women	Sun-exposed skin of the head, neck, and trunk	No identified precursor	Nodular, presenting as a pink or flesh-colored papule, with a "pearly" or translucent quality, and may have visible telangiectasias	Most BCCs remain localized, few become locally aggressive or metastatic
	Superficial (15)	>55 years old Men>Women	Trunk	No identified precursor	Shiny, slightly scaled, pink macule or patch	Typically grow horizontally, but can become invasive
	Infiltrative (5–10)	>65 years old Men>Women	Face	No identified precursor	Pink-to-white, scarlike, indurated papule or plaque, often with atrophic features	These lesions are known for their clinical subtlety and subclinical spread.

		Age	Location	Precursor	Clinical description	Risk
Squamous cell carcinoma	In situ	>45 years old, particularly high in >75 years of age	Sun-exposed skin	No identified precursor, occasionally develop from AKs	Slow-growing, erythematous lesion, with discrete yellow-white scales and dotted vessels	Approximately 2%–5% of cSCC metastasize; considered high risk if >2 cm and very high risk if>4 cm
	Invasive	>45 years old, particularly high in >75 years of age	Sun-exposed skin	No identified precursor, occasionally develop from AKs	Fast-growing, often tender, papule or nodule with a central yellow/white keratin mass and pinpoints of ulceration	Approximately 2%–5% of cSCC metastasize; considered high risk if >2 cm and very high risk if>4 cm
AK	A benign neoplasm	>65 years old	Sun-exposed skin	No identified precursor	Macular lesion with rough texture, scales, and often erythematous	2%–3% of AKs progress to cSCC within 4 years

Abbreviations: AK, actinic keratosis; BCC, basal cell carcinoma; cSCC, cutaneous squamous cell carcinoma; CSD, chronically sun damaged.

many studies have shown an increased risk for melanoma among SOTRs, the relative risk is still much lower than that of KCs.[67] In contrast to the general population, the BCC:SCC ratio for SOTRs is reversed, with significantly higher incidence of cSCC than BCC. This might be explained by a hypothesized co-carcinogen etiology of cSCC that involves both UVR and human papillomavirus (HPV) mutagenesis. Up to 90% of cSCC in SOTRs contain HPV DNA, in contrast to the respective incidence of 11% to 32% in normal skin.[68]

Apart from the contribution of exogenous mutagens, specific *germline mutations* or haplotypes may be associated with increased risk of cSCC in SOTRs.[69] Mutations with the highest associated risk are those among the glutathione S-transferase super-gene family, which combats reactive compounds, such as those produced by UVR. Other common SOTR medications can cause drug-induced alterations associated with increased risk of KC: azathioprine increases 6-thioguanine accumulation in cellular DNA[70,71] and calcineurin inhibitors have also been associated with increased proinflammatory cytokine expression.[72-75]

Protein and messenger RNA *expression profiles* differ among cSCC of SOTRs. Studies that compare cSCC in SOTRs and immunocompetent patients identified 50 unique proteins differentially expressed in SOTRs, including markers of growth and proliferation, anti-apoptotic proteins, DNA repair proteins, immune cell markers, and microRNAs.[69] The latter plays an important role in tumorigenesis, through dysregulation of gene expression and promotion of tumor suppression and growth.[76] Epigenetic alterations are also associated with disparate expression profiles, with hypomethylation and hypermethylation associated with cutaneous cancers.[77,78] These data hold promise for risk stratification and future therapeutic targets.

SKIN CANCER DETECTION AND CURRENT SCREENING RECOMMENDATIONS

Cancer screening practices for providers who are not trained in dermatology are often guided by the US Preventive Services Task Force, which states that current evidence is "insufficient" to evaluate the risk and harms of screening asymptomatic adults for skin cancer.[79] At a societal level, most melanoma screening efforts to date have screened any adult patient who desired screening, a cohort shown to have overall low melanoma incidence. Targeted diagnostic examinations, lesion-directed evaluation of a specific skin growth of concern as identified by the patient or the patient's provider, are an alternative approach. When compared to total body examinations in population-based screening studies, targeted diagnostic examinations detect similar rates of skin cancer and are often less time consuming.[80]

Clinicians with an expert level proficiency in interpreting dermoscopic images of skin growths biopsy fewer benign nevi to diagnose 1 melanoma.[81] Training in dermoscopic image interpretation extends beyond dermatologists: primary care providers (PCPs) frequently address skin concerns and are an important resource for skin cancer detection. Multi-modal training interventions are successful in supporting PCPs in incorporating dermoscopy into clinical practice,[82-84] and a recent consensus statement defines the expected dermoscopic proficiencies for PCPs.[85]

Throughout this review, the authors have discussed common precursors, early-stage lesions, and trajectories of various skin cancers. To aid in detection efforts, these characteristics are summarized in **Table 1**.

SUMMARY

Despite characterizing the molecular landscape of benign, precancerous, and invasive skin cancer lesions, the sequence of genetic alterations that lead to invasive cancer is still not completely understood and precancerous lesions are not precisely defined. The latter is of particular significance, as premalignant lesions show high heterogeneity and genetic variations across cancer subtypes. Subsequently, it's expected that future definitions of precancerous lesions will be molecularly based, rather than histopathologically based.[86] Any aspirations for developing such a molecular-based system will require defining which lesions progress and which enter a state of equilibrium—a process that will require serial tissue biopsies from an evolving lesion, to define the molecular and pathologic features that accurately characterize a precancerous lesion. Extensive characterization of these lesions can improve diagnosis and yield biomarkers that will enable prognostication and allow the determination of lesions that will progress. Ultimately, a comprehensive understanding of the mechanisms by which normal tissues progress to malignant is fundamental for risk stratification and early detection to prevent and treat cancer.

CLINICS CARE POINTS

- Skin cancer initiation and progression are multifactorial and influenced by host and environmental factors, all of which should be considered in the development of treatment and prevention strategies.
- Melanoma arising on non-CSD skin typically occurs at a younger age and follows a pagetoid/superficial growth pattern with slow, horizontal growth and asymmetric border.
- Melanoma arising on CSD skin typically develops de novo and follows a lentiginous growth pattern, clinically presenting as gradually enlarging dark areas on the head and neck of elderly patients.
- NM is an invasive and rapidly growing tumor, arising de novo, and following either non-CSD–associated or CSD-associated patterns.
- DN have a higher mutational burden and distinct mutational pattern than common nevi (CN), yet the risk of an individual DN serving as a precursor lesion to melanoma is similarly low to that of a CN. The presence of DN is associated with an overall increased risk of melanoma development.
- Most cSCCs arise de novo, but the presence of AKs predicts future cSCC development.
- BCC is the most common skin cancer in immunocompetent individuals. BCCs have no identifiable precursor lesions, but early detection can reduce morbidity from locally destructive spread.
- The suppression of immune control is a main factor of tumor initiation and metastasis, and immunosuppression is an important risk factor for all skin cancers.

DISCLOSURE

F. Dimitriou is supported by the Walter and Gertrud Siegenthaler Foundation and the Foundation of University of Zurich, Switzerland.

REFERENCES

1. Kim Y-S, Shin S, Jung SH, et al. Genomic progression of precancerous actinic keratosis to squamous cell carcinoma. J Invest Dermatol 2022;142(3):528–38.e8.
2. Balmain A, Ramsden M, Bowden GT, et al. Activation of the mouse cellular Harvey- ras gene in chemically induced benign skin papillomas. Nature (London) 1984;307(5952):658–60.

3. Cohen C, Zavala-Pompa A, Sequeira JH, et al. Mitogen-actived protein kinase activation is an early event in melanoma progression. Clin Cancer Res 2002; 8(12):3728–33.

4. Schadendorf D, Fisher DE, Garbe C, et al. Melanoma. Nat Rev Dis Prim 2015; 1(1):15003.

5. Rouse J, Jackson SP. Interfaces between the detection, signaling, and repair of DNA damage. Science (American Association for the Advancement of Science) 2002;297(5581):547–51.

6. Maser RS, DePinho RA. Connecting chromosomes, crisis, and cancer. Science (American Association for the Advancement of Science) 2002;297(5581):565–9.

7. Friedberg EC. How nucleotide excision repair protects against cancer. Nat Rev Cancer 2001;1(1):22–33.

8. Hanahan D. Hallmarks of cancer: new dimensions. Cancer Discov 2022;12(1): 31–46.

9. Hanahan D, Coussens LM. Accessories to the crime: functions of cells recruited to the tumor microenvironment. Cancer Cell 2012;21(3):309–22.

10. Huber R, Meier B, Otsuka A, et al. Tumour hypoxia promotes melanoma growth and metastasis via High Mobility Group Box-1 and M2-like macrophages. Sci Rep 2016;6(1):29914.

11. Thomas S, Izard J, Walsh E, et al. The host microbiome regulates and maintains human health: a primer and perspective for non-microbiologists. Cancer Res 2017;77(8):1783–812.

12. Halsey T, Ologun G, Wargo J, et al. Uncovering the role of the gut microbiota in immune checkpoint blockade therapy: A mini-review. Semin Hematol 2020; 57(1):13–8.

13. Spencer CN, McQuade JL, Gopalakrishnan V, et al. Dietary fiber and probiotics influence the gut microbiome and melanoma immunotherapy response. Science (American Association for the Advancement of Science) 2021;374(6575): 1632–40.

14. Witt RG, Cass SH, Tran T, et al. Gut microbiome in patients with early-stage and late-stage melanoma. Arch Dermatol (1960) 2023;159(10):1076–84.

15. Nejman D, Livyatan I, Fuks G, et al. The human tumor microbiome is composed of tumor type-specific intracellular bacteria. Science (American Association for the Advancement of Science) 2020;368(6494):973–80.

16. Maddipati R, Stanger BZ. Pancreatic cancer metastases harbor evidence of polyclonality. Cancer Discov 2015;5(10):1086–97.

17. Sanborn JZ, Chung J, Purdom E, et al. Phylogenetic analyses of melanoma reveal complex patterns of metastatic dissemination. Proceedings of the National Academy of Sciences - PNAS 2015;112(35):10995–1000.

18. Raghavan SS, Kapler ES, Dinges MM, et al. Eruptive Spitz nevus, a striking example of benign metastasis. Sci Rep 2020;10(1):16216.

19. Guy GP, Thomas CC, Thompson T, et al. Vital signs: melanoma incidence and mortality trends and projections — United States, 1982–2030. MMWR. Morbidity and Mortality Weekly report 2015;64(21):591–6.

20. SEER cancer stat facts: melanoma of the skin. national cancer institute. Bethesda, MD, Available at: https://seer.cancer.gov/statfacts/html/melan.html. Accessed September 7, 2023.

21. Tang J, Fewings E, Chang D, et al. The genomic landscapes of individual melanocytes from human skin. Nature (London) 2020;586(7830):600–5.

22. Bastian BC. The molecular pathology of melanoma: an integrated taxonomy of melanocytic neoplasia. Annual Review of Pathology 2014;9(1):239–71.

23. Shain AH, Bastian BC. From melanocytes to melanomas. Nat Rev Cancer 2016; 16(6):345–58.

24. Bevona C, Goggins W, Quinn T, et al. Cutaneous melanomas associated with nevi. Arch Dermatol (1960) 2003;139(12):1620–4.

25. Viros A, Fridlyand J, Bauer J, et al. Improving melanoma classification by integrating genetic and morphologic features. PLoS Med 2008;5(6):e120.

26. Yeh I, Von Deimling A, Bastian BC. Clonal BRAF mutations in melanocytic nevi and initiating role of BRAF in melanocytic neoplasia. J Natl Cancer Inst : J Natl Cancer Inst 2013;105(12):917–9.

27. Patton EE, Widlund HR, Kutok JL, et al. BRAF mutations are sufficient to promote nevi formation and cooperate with p53 in the genesis of melanoma. Curr Biol 2005;15(3):249–54.

28. Tsao H, Bevona C, Goggins W, et al. The transformation rate of moles (Melanocytic Nevi) into cutaneous melanoma: a population-based estimate. Arch Dermatol (1960) 2003;139(3):282–8.

29. Shain AH, Yeh I, Kovalyshyn I, et al. The genetic evolution of melanoma from precursor lesions. N Engl J Med 2015;373(20):1926–36.

30. Krauthammer M, Kong Y, Ha BH, et al. Exome sequencing identifies recurrent somatic RAC1 mutations in melanoma. Nat Genet 2012;44(9):1006–14.

31. Clark JWH, Mihm JMC. Lentigo maligna and lentigo-maligna melanoma. Am J Pathol 1969;55(1):39–67.

32. Weinstock MA, Sober AJ. The risk of progression of lentigo maligna to lentigo maligna melanoma. Br J Dermatol 1987;116(3):303–10.

33. Koh HK, Michalik E, Sober AJ, et al. Lentigo maligna melanoma has no better prognosis than other types of melanoma. J Clin Oncol 1984;2(9):994–1001.

34. Curtin JA, Fridlyand J, Kageshita T, et al. Distinct Sets of Genetic Alterations in Melanoma. N Engl J Med 2005;353(20):2135–47.

35. Massi D, Carli P, Franchi A, et al. Naevus-associated melanomas: cause or chance? Melanoma Res 1999;9(1):85–91.

36. Serrano M, Lin AW, McCurrach ME, et al. Oncogenic ras provokes premature cell senescence associated with accumulation of p53 and p16INK4a. Cell 1997; 88(5):593–602.

37. Freedberg DE, Rigas SH, Russak J, et al. Frequent p16-Independent Inactivation of p14ARF in Human Melanoma. J Natl Cancer Inst 2008;100(11):784–95.

38. Lorbeer FK, Rieser G, Goel A, et al. Distinct senescence mechanisms restrain progression of dysplastic nevi. bioRxiv 2023;07(14):548818.

39. Halpern AC, Guerry D, Elder DE, et al. A cohort study of melanoma in patients with dysplastic nevi. J Invest Dermatol 1993;100(3):S346–9.

40. Gandini S, Sera F, Cattaruzza MS, et al. Meta-analysis of risk factors for cutaneous melanoma: I. Common and atypical naevi. European Journal of Cancer (1990) 2005;41(1):28–44.

41. Rogers HW, Weinstock MA, Feldman SR, et al. Incidence estimate of nonmelanoma skin cancer (keratinocyte carcinomas) in the US population, 2012. JAMA Dermatology (Chicago, Ill.) 2015;151(10):1081–6.

42. Guy GP, Ekwueme DU. Years of potential life lost and indirect costs of melanoma and non-melanoma skin cancer: a systematic review of the literature. Pharmacoeconomics 2011;29(10):863–74.

43. Karia PSMPH, Han JP, Schmults CDMDM. Cutaneous squamous cell carcinoma: Estimated incidence of disease, nodal metastasis, and deaths from disease in the United States, 2012. J Am Acad Dermatol 2013;68(6):957–66.

44. Yilmaz AS, Ozer HG, Gillespie JL, et al. Differential mutation frequencies in met-astatic cutaneous squamous cell carcinomas versus primary tumors. Cancer 2017;123(7):1184–93.
45. Yarchoan M, Hopkins A, Jaffee EM. Tumor mutational burden and response rate to PD-1 inhibition. N Engl J Med 2017;377(25):2500–1.
46. Navsaria LJ, Li Y, Nowakowska MK, et al. Incidence and treatment of actinic kera-tosis in older adults with medicare coverage. Arch Dermatol 2022;158(9):1076–8.
47. Werner RN, Sammain A, Erdmann R, et al. The natural history of actinic keratosis: a systematic review. Br J Dermatol (1951) 2013;169(3):502–18.
48. Marks R, Rennie G, Selwood T. Malignant transformation of solar keratoses to squamous cell carcinoma. Lancet (British edition) 1988;331(8589):795–7.
49. Criscione VD, Weinstock MA, Naylor MF, et al. Actinic keratoses: natural history and risk of malignant transformation in the veterans affairs topical tretinoin che-moprevention trial. Cancer 2009;115(11):2523–30.
50. Zalaudek IMD, Giacomel J, Schmid K, et al. Dermatoscopy of facial actinic kera-tosis, intraepidermal carcinoma, and invasive squamous cell carcinoma: A pro-gression model. J Am Acad Dermatol 2012;66(4):589–97.
51. Pan YM, Chamberlain AJ, Bailey M, et al. Dermatoscopy aids in the diagnosis of the solitary red scaly patch or plaque–features distinguishing superficial basal cell carcinoma, intraepidermal carcinoma, and psoriasis. J Am Acad Dermatol 2008;59(2):268–74.
52. Gailani MR, Ståhle-Bäckdahl M, Leffell DJ, et al. The role of the human homo-logue of Drosophila patched in sporadic basal cell carcinomas. Nat Genet 1996;14(1):78.
53. Altaba ARi, Lee J, Robins P, et al. Activation of the transcription factor Gli1 and the Sonic hedgehog signalling pathway in skin tumours. Nature (London) 1997; 389(6653):876–81.
54. Jr EHE, Murone M, Luoh SM, et al. Activating Smoothened mutations in sporadic basal-cell carcinoma. Nature (London) 1998;391(6662):90–2.
55. Box NF, Duffy DL, Irving RE, et al. Melanocortin-1 Receptor Genotype is a Risk Factor for Basal and Squamous Cell Carcinoma. J Invest Dermatol 2001; 116(2):224–9.
56. Gurzau E, Sulem P, Stacey SN, et al. ASIP and TYR pigmentation variants asso-ciate with cutaneous melanoma and basal cell carcinoma. Nat Genet 2008;40(7): 886–91.
57. Welsh MM, Applebaum KM, Spencer SK, et al. CTLA4 Variants, UV-Induced Tolerance, and Risk of Non-Melanoma Skin Cancer. Cancer research (Chicago, Ill) 2009;69(15):6158–63.
58. Ramachandran S, Lear JT, Ramsay H, et al. Presentation with multiple cutaneous basal cell carcinomas: association of glutathione S-transferase and cytochrome P450 genotypes with clinical phenotype. Cancer Epidemiol Biomarkers Prev 1999;8(1):61.
59. Ramachandran S, Fryer AA, Lovatt TJ, et al. Combined effects of gender, skin type and polymorphic genes on clinical phenotype: use of rate of increase in numbers of basal cell carcinomas as a model system. Cancer Lett 2003; 189(2):175–81.
60. Vesely MD, Schreiber RD. Cancer immunoediting: antigens, mechanisms, and implications to cancer immunotherapy. Ann N Y Acad Sci 2013;1284(1):1–5.
61. Hanahan D, Weinberg Robert A. Hallmarks of cancer: the next generation. Cell 2011;144(5):646–74.

62. Euvrard S, Kanitakis J, Claudy A. Skin cancers after organ transplantation. N Engl J Med 2003;348(17):1681–91.

63. Vajdic CM, van Leeuwen MT. Cancer incidence and risk factors after solid organ transplantation. Int J Cancer 2009;125(8):1747–54.

64. Greenberg JN, Zwald FO. Management of skin cancer in solid-organ transplant recipients: a multidisciplinary approach: mohs surgery. Dermatol Clin 2011; 29(2):231–41.

65. Buell JF, Gross TG, Woodle ES. Malignancy after transplantation. Transplantation 2005;80(2 Suppl):S254–64.

66. Opelz G, Henderson R. Incidence of non-hodgkin lymphoma in kidney and heart transplant recipients. Lancet (British edition) 1993;342(8886):1514–6.

67. Dinh QQ, Chong AH. Melanoma in organ transplant recipients: The old enemy finds a new battleground. Australas J Dermatol 2007;48(4):199–207.

68. Nindl I, Gottschling M, Stockfleth E. Human papillomaviruses and non-melanoma skin cancer: basic virology and clinical manifestations. Dis Markers 2007;23(4): 247–59.

69. Blue ED, Freeman SC, Lobl MB, et al. Cutaneous squamous cell carcinoma arising in immunosuppressed patients: a systematic review of tumor profiling studies. JID innovations 2022;2(4):100126.

70. O'Donovan P, Perrett CM, Zhang X, et al. Azathioprine and UVA light generate mutagenic oxidative DNA damage. Science (American Association for the Advancement of Science) 2005;309(5742):1871–4.

71. Brem R, Li F, Montaner B, et al. DNA breakage and cell cycle checkpoint abrogation induced by a therapeutic thiopurine and UVA radiation. Oncogene 2010; 29(27):3953–63.

72. Xu J, Walsh SB, Verney ZM, et al. Procarcinogenic effects of cyclosporine A are mediated through the activation of TAK1/TAB1 signaling pathway. Biochem Biophys Res Commun 2011;408(3):363–8.

73. Dziunycz PJ, Lefort K, Wu X, et al. The oncogene ATF3 Is potentiated by cyclosporine A and ultraviolet light A. J Invest Dermatol 2014;134(7):1998–2004.

74. Abikhair M, Mitsui H, Yanofsky V, et al. Cyclosporine A immunosuppression drives catastrophic squamous cell carcinoma through IL-22. JCI Insight 2016;1(8): e86434.

75. Abikhair Burgo M, Roudiani N, Chen J, et al. Ruxolitinib inhibits cyclosporine-induced proliferation of cutaneous squamous cell carcinoma. JCI Insight 2018;3(17).

76. Peng Y, Croce CM. The role of MicroRNAs in human cancer. Signal Transduct Targeted Ther 2016;1(1):15004.

77. Sigalotti L, Coral S, Nardi G, et al. Promoter methylation controls the expression of MAGE2, 3 and 4 genes in human cutaneous melanoma. J Immunother 2002; 25(1):16–26.

78. Tyler LN, Ai L, Zuo C, et al. Analysis of promoter hypermethylation of death-associated protein kinase and p16 tumor suppressor genes in actinic keratoses and squamous cell carcinomas of the skin. Mod Pathol 2003;16(7):660–4.

79. Mangione CM, Mangione CM, Barry MJ, et al. Screening for skin cancer: US preventive services task force recommendation statement. JAMA 2023;329(15): 1290–5.

80. Hoorens I, Vossaert K, Pil L, et al. Total-Body Examination vs Lesion-Directed Skin Cancer Screening. JAMA Dermatol 2016;152(1):27–34.

81. Dinnes J, Deeks JJ, Chuchu N, et al. Dermoscopy, with and without visual inspection, for diagnosing melanoma in adults. Cochrane Database Syst Rev 2018; 2018(12):CD011902.
82. Nelson KC, Seiverling EV, Gonna N, et al. A Pilot educational intervention to support primary care provider performance of skin cancer examinations. J Cancer Educ 2023;38(1):364–9.
83. Seiverling E, Ahrns H, Stevens K, et al. Dermoscopic lotus of learning: implementation and dissemination of a multimodal dermoscopy curriculum for primary care. Journal of Medical Education and Curricular Development 2021;8. 2382120521989983.
84. Seiverling EV, Stevens K, Dorr G, et al. Impact of multimodal dermatoscopy training on skin biopsies by primary care providers. J Am Acad Dermatol 2022; 87(5):1119–21.
85. Tran T, Cyr PR, Verdieck A, et al. Expert consensus statement on proficiency standards for dermoscopy education in primary care. J Am Board Fam Med 2023; 36(1):25–38.
86. Srivastava S, Wagner PD, Hughes SK, et al. Precancer atlas: present and future. Cancer Prevention Research (Philadelphia, Pa.) 2023;16(7):379–84.

Biomarkers in Cancer Screening

Promises and Challenges in Cancer Early Detection

Indu Kohaar, PhD[a], Nicholas A. Hodges, PhD[a],
Sudhir Srivastava, PhD, MPH[a],*

KEYWORDS

- Precancer • Biomarkers • Early detection • Screening

KEY POINTS

- Screening and early detection for clinically significant cancer is key to prevention.
- Defining and characterizing the precancer lesion/state provides an opportunity for early cancer prevention and interception.
- New developments in molecular cancer screening and early detection including well-designed multi-cancer detection trials will pave the way for cancer prevention and reducing the cancer screening and detection-related mortality, morbidity, and associated cost.

INTRODUCTION

Cancer is a major public health and economic burden worldwide with an estimated 19.3 million new cancer cases and 10 million deaths in 2020, approximately accounting for 1 in 6 deaths.[1] In 2023, a total of 1.9 million new cancer cases and 610,000 cancer-related deaths are projected in the USA, indicating slight decrease in the overall cancer mortality.[2] Detecting and treating cancer at early stages enables more effective treatment and reduces morbidity and mortality.[3] 5-year survival rate across all cancers reduces from 89% when localized to 21% once metastasized.[4] For example, in colorectal cancer, the 5-year survival for stage I is 80% to 95%, but it is less than 15% when detected at stage IV. Likewise, the 5-year survival for resectable stage IA pancreatic cancer is about 85%, but less than 10% when detected at an advanced stage.[5,6]

[a] Cancer Biomarkers Research Group, Division of Cancer Prevention, National Cancer Institute, NIH, 9609 Medical Center Drive, NCI Shady Grove Building, Rockville, MD 20850, USA
* Corresponding author.
E-mail address: srivasts@mail.nih.gov

Hematol Oncol Clin N Am 38 (2024) 869–888
https://doi.org/10.1016/j.hoc.2024.04.004
0889-8588/24/Published by Elsevier Inc.
hemonc.theclinics.com

Although there is inconclusive evidence that prostate-specific antigen (PSA)-based screening results in a decrease in prostate cancer (PCa) mortality,[7-10] early detection has resulted in significant increase in the number of men diagnosed with localized and locally advanced disease. Since 2014, PCa incidence has increased by 3%/year, mostly driven by 4% to 5%/year increase in incidence of regional and distant stage diagnosis.[11] Randomized clinical trials (RCTs) investigating PSA-screening have demonstrated a reduction in the incidence of de novo metastatic PCa, but this has not been studied in large, population-based studies.[12]

Additionally, costs associated with treating cancers diagnosed at a late-stage are up to 7 times higher than those diagnosed at an early-stage, leading to significant economic burden.[2] Early detection includes early diagnosis and screening. According to the Unites States Preventive Task Force (USPSTF), single-site cancer screening is recommended for colorectal, breast, cervical, and lung cancer for at-risk individuals (**Fig. 1**).[13-17] Early cancer detection through established screening/diagnostic approaches has now led to cervical, breast, and colorectal cancers being diagnosed sooner, at earlier stages, than cancers without established screening modalities, which constitute almost 70% of the cancer deaths in US.[2] Many cancers such as pancreatic, esophageal, and ovarian cancers are often diagnosed at advanced stages leading to significant morbidity and mortality.

Thus, there is a critical need to identify cancer specific biomarkers which in conjunction with imaging methods can improve screening/diagnosis of cancers with no

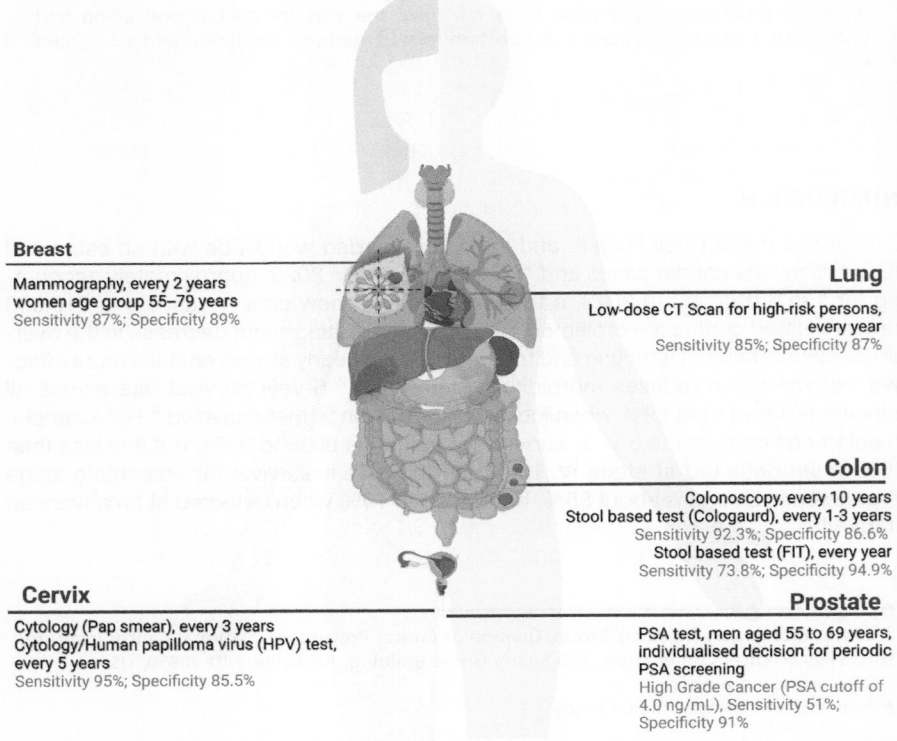

Breast

Mammography, every 2 years
women age group 55–79 years
Sensitivity 87%; Specificity 89%

Lung

Low-dose CT Scan for high-risk persons,
every year
Sensitivity 85%; Specificity 87%

Colon

Colonoscopy, every 10 years
Stool based test (Cologaurd), every 1-3 years
Sensitivity 92.3%; Specificity 86.6%
Stool based test (FIT), every year
Sensitivity 73.8%; Specificity 94.9%

Cervix

Cytology (Pap smear), every 3 years
Cytology/Human papilloma virus (HPV) test,
every 5 years
Sensitivity 95%; Specificity 85.5%

Prostate

PSA test, men aged 55 to 69 years,
individualised decision for periodic
PSA screening
High Grade Cancer (PSA cutoff of
4.0 ng/mL), Sensitivity 51%;
Specificity 91%

Fig. 1. USPSTF—recommended screening tests for cancer. USPSTF, United States preventive Services Taskforce. (Created with BioRender.com.)

established standard of care method. The need for continued research also persists for those cancers where the currently available biomarkers do not have optimal clinical performance like the PSA test for prostate cancer. According to the National Cancer Institute (NCI), a biomarker is "a biological molecule found in blood, other body fluids, or tissues that is a sign of a normal or abnormal process, or of a condition or disease"[18] and are objectively measured and evaluated as an indicator of normal biological processes, pathogenic processes, or pharmacologic responses to a therapeutic intervention.[19] The rationale for selecting a biomarker in the cancer field includes its ability for predicting risk, early detection, staging, monitoring treatment response, and tracking disease progression. This is in addition to a biomarkers ability to reduce overdiagnosis, distinguish aggressive from non-aggressive lesion types, and inform selection of patients for specific treatment options, thereby leading to greater life expectancy and quality of life for the patient.[20] The characteristics of an ideal biomarker are high specificity, sensitivity, quantifiability, ease-of-use, reproducibility, clear and concise read-outs for clinicians, cost-effectiveness, and can be measured from easily acquired biological fluid or specimen. The present review primarily addresses the current state of knowledge of available early detection molecular markers in cancer, new developments and technologies in the field, and discusses their challenges and potential for clinical utility. Imaging modalities are not discussed here.

CURRENT SCREENING AND EARLY DETECTION MODALITIES

We have used the phrases "early detection" and "screening" interchangeably. However, screening is a process involving multiple modalities, e.g., biomarkers, imaging, and so forth that looks for cancer before symptoms appear. Early detection, on the other hand, looks for the earliest stage of disease that is clinically manageable. Screening is improved for cancers with an established early asymptomatic phase and available clinically validated, safe, sensitive, specific, and straightforward screening test with strong patient adherence, acceptance by patients and clinicians, and cost effectiveness.

USPSTF recommended screening tests for breast, colon, lung, prostate, and cervical cancers along with their clinical performance is shown in **Fig. 1**. Screening is more effective for slow growing tumors than rapidly growing tumors due to lead-time bias. Yet, screening suffers from overdiagnosis of certain cancers, leading to overtreatment or unnecessary diagnostic biopsy procedures. Further, in relation to the clinical performance, most of the screening tests have sensitivity and specificity in ranges of 70% to 80% and 60% to 70% respectively,[21] low positive predictive value (PPV)[22,23] and high overall false positive rate when the test is used sequentially[24] and therefore is not a perfect solution to early detection. Additionally, there is bias effect of disease prevalence on PPV; for cervical cancer with disease prevalence of less than 0.1%, PPV is less than 0.1%, while for high-risk lung cancer with disease prevalence of 1.1%, PPV is 6.9%. Other limitations are compliance with recommended screening tests for example, compliance is in range of 69% to 80% for breast, cervical, and colorectal cancers while it is 5% for lung cancer[25–29] and lower cancer screening rate within underrepresented racial/ethnic populations.[2,30] Additionally, biological and technical challenges of endogenous markers including tumor heterogeneity, interpatient variation, comorbidities, and background signal by healthy cells, remain obstacles for the early detection of cancer specially before the symptoms appear.[31] Therefore, we must explore new multi-analyte tests which incorporate new quantitative imaging modalities with adjunct biomarker/screening assays, which can be broadly applied across patients with different ancestries.

TYPES OF EARLY LESIONS

In response to the Cancer Moonshot Initiative's Blue-Ribbon Panel recommendation, NCI launched the Human Tumor Atlas Network (HTAN) program with the overall goal of generation of human tumor atlases. The results of this initiative are helping toward defining the precancer framework, which should be dynamic and adaptable with following important interrelated components: histopathological features, biology in conjunction with disease outcome, changes in the precancer microenvironment, and molecular features derived from the integration of the multi-omics data.[32] Precancerous lesions are high-risk lesions/states that often lead to the development of invasive carcinoma (**Fig. 2**). These lesions include high-grade dysplasia (HGD) for esophagus, adenoma HGD for colorectum, ductal carcinoma in situ (DCIS) for breast, pancreatic intraepithelial neoplasia (PanIN) for pancreas, prostatic intraepithelial neoplasia for prostate, high-grade squamous intraepithelial lesions/carcinoma-in-situ 3 for cervix, bladder carcinoma in situ/noninvasive papillary carcinoma for bladder, HGD for stomach, Bowen's disease, actinic keratosis (AK), lentigo maligna for skin, squamous carcinoma in situ (CIS) for lung, oral epithelial dysplasia/CIS for mouth, anal intraepithelial lesions for anus, renal intraepithelial lesions for kidney, serous tubular intraepithelial carcinoma for ovary. These lesions can be found in screening procedures of high-risk patients or using diagnostic biopsies in patients suspicious of cancer or in cases of incidental cancer. Precancers for hematologic conditions include monoclonal B-cell lymphocytosis for chronic lymphocytic leukemia and monoclonal gammopathy of undetermined significance/smoldering myeloma for myeloma. Although precancerous lesions are common in general population for

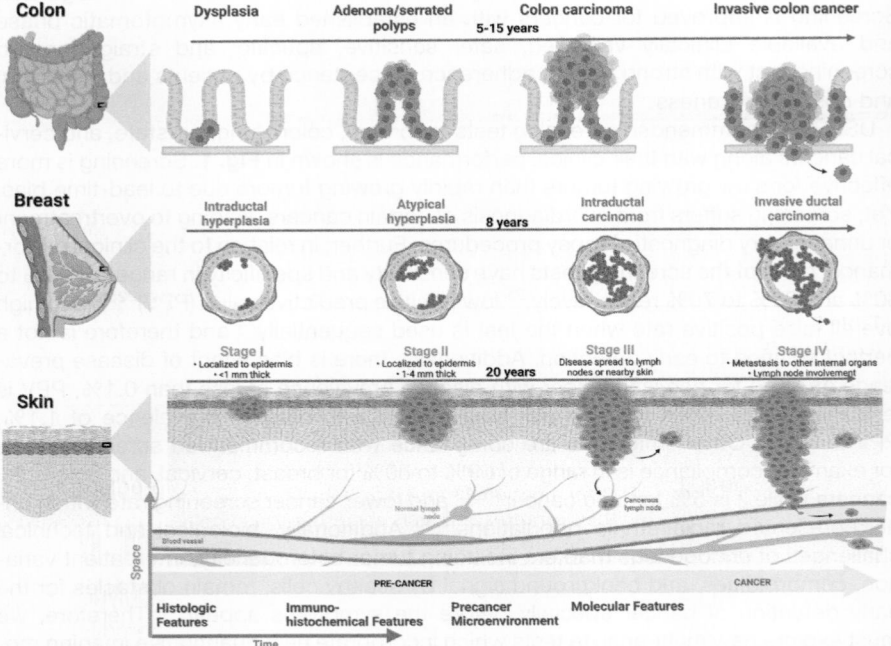

Fig. 2. Examples of early lesions and transition to invasive cancer. (Created with BioRender. com.)

certain types (example-10% in breast biopsies,[33] 24% in colon polyps,[34] 43% in pancreatic intra-epithelial neoplasia [PanIN1],[35] 49% of AK in men),[36] not all precancerous cells progress into cancer.[37,38] It was found that 20% of breast precancer,[39] 15% to 25% of colon polyps,[40] 10% to 15% of PanIN,[41] and 10% of AK lesions[42] progress to invasive stages. Additionally, there is a long transition period from development of precancer to invasive cancer which can span from 5 to 15 years for colorectal,[34] 8 years for breast,[33] 25 to 30 years for skin,[36] and more than 10 years for prostate cancers,[43] with exceptions for lung (2 years)[44] and pancreatic cancers (5 years).[45] However, the higher likelihood of progression from precancerous stage to aggressive form of cancer in many cases implies that it is important to have an accurate, objective, and easy-to-use method/biomarker to identify critical initial events leading to aggressive premalignant lesions from normal. Although the histopathological progression of these lesions has been well characterized for many cancers, there is still a dearth of information on key molecular events leading the transition of precancerous lesions to aggressive, invasive cancer. New HTAN pre-cancer atlas (PCA) initiative has started shedding light on comprehensive understanding of the molecular, cellular, and tissue alterations and the interactions of the various cell types that drive tumor development and progression, especially the progression from premalignant lesions to invasive cancer. For example, spatial PCA of breast cancer revealed that when normal breast specimens with patient-matched DCIS and invasive breast cancer (IBC) were compared, distinct coordinated transitions in their tumor microenvironment (TME) were observed. Interestingly, myoepithelial disruption was more advanced in patients with DCIS that did not develop IBC, implying this process could be protective against recurrence by allowing immune infiltration.[46,47] Thus, the findings from HTAN PCA research efforts could have implication on improvements in risk stratification, early detection, and development of cancer prevention/interception strategies. NCI's 2023 PCA initiative will address this need by developing comprehensive, dynamic, high-resolution, multidimensional, multiparametric, and scalable atlases of precancerous lesions and their surrounding microenvironment.[48]

EARLY DETECTION BIOMARKERS

Early detection biomarkers refer to the genomic, epigenomic, proteomic, metabolic, and metabolomic molecules derived from human specimens (blood, urine, saliva, tumor, and so forth.) that inform risk and diagnosis for a disease/cancer.[49] Biomarkers of risk include hereditary cancers where the patients have germline predisposition to certain cancers. Some examples of such cancers/hereditary cancer syndromes (with associated germline mutations in gene) include hereditary non-polyposis colon cancer (DNA mismatch repair genes *MLH1*, *MSH2*, *MSH6* or *PMS2*), hereditary breast and ovarian cancer (*BRCA1*, *BRCA2*), familial adenomatous polyposis, Li-Fraumeni Syndrome (*TP53*), Cowden Syndrome (*PTEN*), and Von Hippel-Lindau disease. Diagnostic biomarkers include markers, which are either abnormal or/and are elevated in body fluids, which can provide information on the course of the disease. **Table 1** lists commonly used diagnostic tumor markers for cancer that may have additional clinical utility in relation to disease management.

NEW DEVELOPMENTS IN MOLECULAR CANCER SCREENING AND EARLY DETECTION
Germline Testing

Nearly 10% of all cancers are caused by inherited genetic changes/germline mutations in cancer susceptibility genes.[50] Expanding the National Comprehensive Cancer Network clinical practice guidelines in oncology (NCCN Guidelines): on recommendations of

Table 1
Common use early detection tumor markers

	Cancer Type	Specimen Type	Clinical Utility
Alpha-fetoprotein (AFP)	Liver cancer	Blood	Diagnosis, treatment response
B-cell immunoglobulin gene rearrangement	B-cell lymphoma	Blood, bone marrow, or tumor tissue	Diagnosis, treatment response, check for recurrence
BCL2 gene rearrangement	Lymphomas, leukemias	Blood, bone marrow, or tumor tissue	Diagnosis, treatment determination
Beta-human chorionic gonadotropin (Beta-hCG)	Choriocarcinoma and germ cell tumors	Urine or blood	Stage assessment, prognosis, treatment response
Bladder tumor antigen (BTA)	Bladder cancer and cancer of the kidney or ureter	Urine	Diagnosis, check for recurrence
BCR-ABL fusion gene (Philadelphia chromosome)	Chronic myeloid leukemia, acute lymphoblastic leukemia, and acute myelogenous leukemia	Blood or bone marrow	Diagnosis, treatment determination, monitor disease status, treatment response
BRCA1 and BRCA2	Breast, ovarian, and cervical cancers	Blood or saliva	Diagnosis, treatment determination
C-kit/CD117	Gastrointestinal stromal tumor, mucosal melanoma, acute myeloid leukemia, and mast cell disease	Tumor, blood, or bone marrow	Diagnosis, treatment determination
CA-125	Ovarian cancer	Blood	Diagnosis, treatment response, check for recurrence
Calcitonin	Medullary thyroid cancer	Blood	Diagnosis, treatment response, check for recurrence
CD19	B-cell lymphomas and leukemias	Blood and bone marrow	Diagnosis, treatment determination
CD22	B-cell lymphomas and leukemias	Blood and bone marrow	Diagnosis, treatment determination

Biomarker	Cancer / condition	Sample	Clinical use
Chromogranin A (CgA)	Neuroendocrine tumors	Blood	Diagnosis, treatment response, check for recurrence
Cyclin D1 (CCND1) gene rearrangement or expression	Lymphoma, myeloma	Tumor	Diagnosis
DNA mismatch repair genes (MSH2, MLH1, MSH6, PSM2)	Lynch syndrome (colon cancer)	Blood or saliva	Diagnosis
Gastrin	Gastrin-producing tumor (gastrinoma)	Blood	Diagnosis, treatment response, check for recurrence
5-HIAA	Carcinoid tumors	Urine	Diagnosis and disease monitoring
Human papilloma virus (HPV)	Cervical cancer	Cervical cells	Diagnosis
Immunoglobulins	Multiple myeloma and Waldenström macroglobulinemia	Blood and urine	Diagnosis, treatment response, check for recurrence
IRF4 gene rearrangement	Lymphoma	Tumor	Diagnosis
JAK2 gene mutation	Certain types of leukemia	Blood and bone marrow	Diagnosis
KIT gene (KIT)	Gastrointestinal stromal tumors	Tumor	Diagnosis, prognosis
Microsatellite instability (MSI) and/ or mismatch repair deficient (dMMR)	Colorectal cancer and other solid tumors	Tumor	Identify those at high risk of certain cancer-predisposing syndromes, treatment determination
MYC gene expression	Lymphomas, leukemias	Tumor	Diagnosis, treatment determination
MYD88 gene mutation	Lymphoma, Waldenström macroglobulinemia	Tumor	Diagnosis, treatment determination
Myeloperoxidase (MPO)	Leukemia	Blood	Diagnosis
Neuron-specific enolase (NSE)	Small cell lung cancer and neuroblastoma	Blood	Diagnosis, treatment response,
PCA3 mRNA	Prostate cancer	Urine (collected after digital rectal exam)	Diagnosis (repeat biopsy after negative biopsy)

(continued on next page)

Table 1
(continued)

	Cancer Type	Specimen Type	Clinical Utility
PML/RARα fusion gene	Acute promyelocytic leukemia (APL)	Blood and bone marrow	Diagnosis, treatment determination, monitor disease status, treatment response
Prostatic acid phosphatase (PAP)	Metastatic prostate cancer	Blood	Diagnosis for poorly differentiated carcinomas
Prostate-specific antigen (PSA)	Prostate cancer	Blood	Diagnosis, treatment response, check for recurrence
T-cell receptor gene rearrangement	T-cell lymphoma	Bone marrow, tissue, body fluid, blood	Diagnosis; detection and evaluation of residual disease
Terminal transferase (TdT)	Leukemia, lymphoma	Tumor, blood	Diagnosis
Urine catecholamines: VMA and HVA	Neuroblastoma	Urine	Diagnosis
FoundationOne CDx (F1CDx) genomic test	Any solid tumor	Tumor, blood	Companion diagnostic test to determine treatment
Guardant360 CDx genomic test	Any solid tumor	Blood	Companion diagnostic test to determine treatment; general tumor mutation profiling
5-Protein signature (OVA1)	Ovarian cancer	Blood	To pre-operatively assess pelvic mass for suspected ovarian cancer

National Cancer Institute.Tumor Marker Tests in Common Use. December 7, 2023. Available at: https://www.cancer.gov/about-cancer/diagnosis-staging/diagnosis/tumor-markers-list.

genetic testing to assess risk and management of hereditary cancers, including ovarian, breast, endometrial, colorectal cancers, and pancreatic cancers reveals the increased importance of germline testing in cancer prevention, risk, and treatment.[51] Currently, genetic testing involves screening for pathogenic/likely pathogenic (P/LP) germline variants in cancer predisposition genes including BRCA1, BRCA2, CDH1, PALB2, PTEN, and TP53 which are associated with increased risk of breast, colorectal, ovarian, pancreatic, and prostate cancer. It also provides recommended measures for genetic counseling/testing and management strategies for individuals carrying P/LP germline variants. It has been found that germline mutations in BRCA1 and BRCA2 result in an increased risk for developing breast and ovarian cancer.[52] The patients carrying P/LP germline variants in BRCA1/2 have an increased risk of developing cancer at an early age and have risk of multiple primary cancers. Lynch syndrome is an autosomal dominant genetic disease caused by germline mutations in DNA mismatch repair genes (MLH1, MSH2, MSH6, and PMS2). This cancer syndrome is associated with high risk of colon and endometrial cancers, accounting for about 1% to 3% of all colorectal cancer cases and 2% to 3% of all endometrial cancer cases.[53]

Recently, for the first time the U.S. Food and Drug Administration (FDA) granted marketing authorization to the Invitae Common Hereditary Cancers Panel, which is an in vitro next-generation sequencing based diagnostic test that can identify germline variants in 47 cancer predisposing genes associated with an elevated risk of developing certain types of cancer.[54] The Invitae panel includes BRCA1 and BRCA2, Lynch syndrome associated genes (MLH1, MSH2, MSH6, PMS2 and EPCAM), CDH1 (mainly associated with hereditary diffuse gastric cancer and lobular breast cancer), and STK11 (linked with Peutz-Jeghers Syndrome). However, the challenges of incorporating germline testing in the clinical workflow are lack of clarity on the approach (targeted or universal gene panel testing), lack of knowledge of the clinical performance of the assays in racially diverse individuals, and absence of standardized systems for implementation in the clinic.

Synthetic Biomarkers

Nanoparticles are a class of synthetic biomarkers that represent a novel approach in the field of medical diagnostics and personalized medicine. Nanoparticles are designed to specifically recognize and interact with molecular targets, such as proteins, nucleic acids, lipids, or metabolites. While traditional biomarkers are limited by dilution and signal-to-noise ratio, nanoparticles can be artificially designed to activate or enhance expression and track progression of precancerous lesions. One such method is attaching reporter molecules to particles larger than the filtration limit of kidneys (> 8 nm). Otherwise undetectable tumor-secreted protease activity can be measured in urine samples after cleaving detectable markers from injected particles.[55–57] These particles can be developed into a multicancer biosensor by attaching multiple reporters that provide a complex overview of precancerous and cancerous progression and activity.[58,59] Synthetic cleavable reporters can also be attached to an enzyme substrate to form small molecule probes that directly target metabolic pathways,[60] reactive oxygen species,[61] or volatile organic compounds.[62] Gold nanoparticles (AuNPs) have extensive uses in imaging technology due to their unique physical, chemical, and electronic properties. In addition, AuNPs spontaneously accumulate a serum protein corona to reduce surface energy that can be used to characterize the circulating serum proteins.[63] These nanoparticle-enabled blood tests of pancreatic ductal adenocarcinoma (PDAC) patient plasma have shown promise in detection both in specificity and sensitivity.[64] The protein corona can be formed before application to stabilize molecular probes to the particles. Wu and colleagues utilized the protein corona of gold nanoclusters to stabilize fluorescent polystyrene nanoparticles conjugated to epithelial cell adhesion molecule (EpCAM) aptamer to detect breast cancer cells *in vitro* and *in vivo* in mice.[65] Although nanoparticle use in early detection seems promising, the risks and adverse effects for infusion of nanomaterials are unknown.

Quantum dots (QDs) are a subset of nanoparticles consisting of semiconductor nanocrystals whose small size (2–10 nm) enable quantum mechanical properties. Within nanoscale semiconductors, a stimulus causes an electron to cross the band gap from the valence band to the higher energy conduction band; these QDs emit fluorescence when the electron returns to the valence band. The color produced is determined by the wavelength emitted by the band gap which itself is dependent on the size of the particle undergoing excitation.[66] Attaching molecular sensors (antibody, ligand, and so forth.) to QDs allows for studies in cancer biomarker detection, tumor identification, and TME mapping. However, QDs have been limited to mostly in vitro applications due to the potential for heavy metal ion toxicity,[67,68] but recent efforts have been made to reduce toxicity through formulation of carbon[69] and graphene QDs.[70] Carbon dots attached to triaminoguanidine as a receptor for citrate, a potential biomarker for prostate cancer,[71] were able to detect citrate presence in both cell culture and human urine samples with low cytotoxicity.[72] Another challenge for *in vivo* QDs is the need for specificity and imaging that can penetrate to the depth of tumor sites. Liu and colleagues developed a nanosystem of near-infrared QDs equipped with the tumor-penetrating peptide iRGD for a mouse model of pancreatic and orthotopic breast tumors.[73] The QDs were designed to undergo signal quenching through cation exchange to reduce background signal and toxicity through release of metal ions that were cleared renally. Near-infrared imaging identified an accumulation of QDs in fibroblasts and extravascular tumor cells with high specificity. Although iRGD peptide offers promise for improving the *in vivo* tumor imaging in the preclinical models, this approach further warrants investigation with respect to specificity and uptake by non-target cells.

Genetically encoded synthetic biomarkers utilize genetic engineering techniques to integrate within targeted tumor cells or neighboring cells in the TME to detect, report, or respond to molecular signals indicative of cancer. Vector-based biomarkers utilize plasmids or viruses to insert secretable reporters directly into the tumor cells by targeting tumor-specific promoters.[74] An enhanced green fluorescent protein encoding oncolytic herpes simplex virus was used in a human trial of peritoneal cytology in pancreatic cancer to detect micro-metastasis and correlated to patient outcomes.[75] Alternatively, resident cells that target the TME can be engineered to seek a precancerous lesion or tumor and secrete biomarkers for detection. One such study used macrophages that were modified to release Gaussia luciferase (Gluc) when polarized to an M2 tumor-associated macrophage phenotype.[76] Alternatively, bacteria have emerged as a promising vector for genetic biomarkers.[77,78] In a mouse model of colorectal cancer, genetically modified bacteria (A. baylyi) have been programmed to leverage the bacterial horizontal gene transfer capability to develop drug resistance in response to uptake of the mutated *KRAS* gene shed from tumor cells. These bacteria samples were then transferred to an antibiotic selection agar plate to detect *KRAS* mutations.[79]

Although, synthetic biomarkers hold a great promise in detecting cancer early, there are some caveats that need to be addressed in the field including background noise due to off-target and on-target, off-tumor activation, lack of standardized preclinical models for precancer and early-stage cancer, and limited understanding of the biology of early lesions and their transitions into malignancy. Since the field is still in infancy, human testing of synthetic biomarkers in well-designed trials will ultimately determine its utility in early cancer detection.

Liquid Biopsy

The U.S. NCI definition of liquid biopsy is "A laboratory test done on a sample of blood, urine, or other body fluid to look for cancer cells from a tumor or small pieces of DNA, RNA, or other molecules released by tumor cells into a person's body fluids." Liquid biopsy allows multiple samples to be taken over time, which may help doctors understand what kind of genetic or molecular changes are taking place in a tumor. A liquid biopsy may be used to help find cancer at an early stage. It may also be used to help plan treatment or to find out how well treatment is working or if cancer has come back.[80]" Although tissue biopsy is long considered gold standard to diagnose cancer, it only provides a single snapshot of the tumor, suffers from selection bias, and is not reflective of inter and intratumorally heterogeneity.

Additionally, multiple biopsies from the tumor are sometimes performed; this process is limited in relation to the chance of targeting/accessibility of tumor, surgical complications, and associated costs. On the other hand, liquid biopsy is relatively easy to perform, does not have selection bias for the tumor region as opposed to a tumor biopsy and can be used for longitudinal monitoring. Over the past 2 decades, liquid biopsy sources have expanded to include various biofluid specimens including blood, urine, cerebrospinal fluid, saliva, amniotic fluid, ascitic fluid examining cancer-derived circulating tumor cells (CTCs), circulating nucleic acids including cell-free DNA (cfDNA), circulating tumor DNA, cell-free RNA including mRNA, long non-coding RNAs and microRNA (miRNA), extracellular vesicles , tumor-informed platelets, proteins, and metabolites (1, 2). Most of the FDA-approved liquid biopsy tests are prognostic tests including Cell Search Circulating Tumor Cell (CTC) Test, Cobas EGFR Mutation Test v2, Guardant360 CDx, FoundationOne Liquid CDx, and Therascreen PIK3CA Mutation Analysis which aids clinicians to help identify patients with cancer who may benefit from specific FDA-approved treatments.[81] This implies that there is a critical need to develop diagnostic and molecular screening biomarkers in addition to the standard of care methods and to establish their clinical utility in context of precancer or cancer diagnosis and screening.

Microfluidic chips are devices that use small channels to manipulate and control miniscule amounts of fluid on the order of microliters or smaller to simulate the tissue microenvironment. The microchannels function by capillary action that allows the flow of fluids through the microchannels without requiring an external pressure source, but microfluidic platforms can also be powered by pumps or gravity as the design requires.[82] In the context of cancer detection, microfluidic technology offers innovative approaches that enable highly sensitive, rapid, and cost-effective methods for detecting cancer-specific biomarkers, CTCs, and cfDNA from liquid biopsies. The SMILE (SAW-MIP Integrated Device for Oral Cancer Early Detection) platform was developed for point-of-care early screening of oral squamous cell carcinoma (OSCC).[83] The system uses immobilized anti-EpCAM to selectively capture tumor cells before injecting a secondary solution for staining. Other microfluidic systems screen for precancerous and early stage OSCC via changes in the amount and function of salivary cytokines IL-6[84] and IL-8.[85] However, keeping the isolated CTCs affixed to the surface of the device when rinsing remains a challenge particularly in early cancer detection when few CTCs are in circulation. Microchannels lined with AuNPs conjugated to anti-EpCAM irreversibly sequestered CTCs from human blood and improved sensitivity for cancer detection.[86] Cancerous cfDNA from liquid biopsies is heavily diluted with a short half-life therefore extraction requires precision and speed. A pressure and immiscibility based extraction microfluidic chip successfully monitored the progression of HER-2 type breast cancer from plasma cfDNA and recognized a point mutation in phosphatidylinositol-4,5-bisphosphate 3-kinase (PIK3CA) during liver metastasis.[87] To make this technology accessible for point-of-care screening, the device must be scalable to produce while the targeting antibodies must remain functional for extended periods of time. To overcome these restraints, new materials, rather than traditional polydimethylsiloxane (PDMS), provide longer term capability and ease of fabrication.[88,89] Cryodesiccation of microfluidic devices preserves the bioactivity of the attached antibodies and substantially extends the storage time.[90] The implementation of microfluidic-based systems holds considerable potential for improving early diagnosis, monitoring disease progression, and providing cost-effective cancer detection. However, the technology has to be standardized and rigorously validated for efficiency, reproducibility, and potential clinical utility.

Some of these tests are single-organ marker tests for specific cancers like Epi pro-Colon and Bluestar Genomics' 5hmC Assay while other assays are multi-cancer detection (MCD) assays like CancerSeek, Galleri, and OverC MCD Assay. Currently, the only FDA premarket-approved liquid biopsy test being utilized for colorectal screening is the Epi proColon. It is performed by detecting methylated Septin 9 (SEPT9) DNA using blood samples.[91] A multi-institutional study on 1544 patients across Europe and the USA found that Epi proColon achieved a sensitivity of 68% and a specificity of 80% when comparing Epi proColon to colonoscopies for screening of colorectal cancer.[92] The Bluestar Genomics' 5hmC Assay is another test used for pancreatic cancer detection that received the Breakthrough Device designation in 2021. It is a blood-based test which measures the levels of the biomarker 5-hydroxymethylcytosine (5hmC). In a recently completed case-control validation study, the Bluestar Genomics test achieved sensitivity of 67% and specificity of 97% in a population of 2150 patients over the age of 50.[93] PCR screening for cell free EBV DNA in plasma samples for a cohort of 20,174 asymptomatic persons for early nasopharyngeal carcinoma showed positivity for 1.5% of the patients and 0.17% of the patients were found to have nasopharyngeal carcinoma on endoscopic evaluation.[94]

Unlike conventional cancer screening methods that focus on specific types of cancer, MCD tests aim to detect various cancers simultaneously, including more than 60% of cancers that do not have screening in standard of care. Though MCD technology is intended to screen patients that are symptom-free, many of the published studies determining the sensitivity and specificity of MCDs assessed blood plasma from patients whose cancer diagnoses were known prior to the study.[95–97] Cancer-SEEK is one recently developed MCD based on circulating proteins and mutations in cfDNA.[95] The CancerSEEK study of 1005 patients with non-metastatic cancer showed test positivity in a median of 70% of 8 cancer types (ovarian, liver, stomach, pancreatic, esophageal, colorectal, lung, and breast). Overall sensitivity ranged from 69% to 98% with a specificity of greater than 99% for the detection of 5 cancer types (ovary, liver, stomach, pancreas, and esophagus) in average-risk subjects. Further implementation of artificial intelligence (AI) is key to the development of MCDs but requires training data sets from established patient information.[98] The Cell-free Genome Atlas study was a case-controlled, observational study that integrated machine learning with methylation-based cfDNA to detect cancer signals across multiple cancer types with intermediate sensitivity.[99] Though known cancer status is important for validating sensitivity, specificity is required to make MCDs clinically effective. In a study of asymptomatic patients, DETECT-A was a prospective interventional clinical trial to evaluate an MCD blood test that evaluated 9911 women with no history of cancer.[100] Positive tests were independently verified by PET-CT scans determining a high specificity (>99%) with 1% false positives and 65% of cancers were detected at an early stage, with sensitivity varying with the tumor type. In an ongoing prospective clinical trial, ASCEND is validating a classification algorithm for a new version of the CancerSEEK assay utilizing 1000 patients with diagnosed/suspected cancer and 2000 patients with unknown cancer status. Additional GRAIL MCD trials intended for use in screening asymptomatic populations include STRIVE, SUMMIT, PATHFINDER, and the GRAIL/UK NHS partnership.[101,102]

While determining cancer risk is the general goal of MCD, the greater diagnostic consideration is a tissue-of-origin (TOO) for the most likely organ for cancer development. Most of the TOO algorithms are proprietary and a black box. However, based on the published literature, circulating miRNA appears to be a prime candidate for TOO determination for MCDs.[103,104] Recent studies have taken a predictive model of miRNAnomics for stage 1 lung cancer and expanded to biliary tract, bladder, colorectal, esophageal, gastric, glioma, liver, pancreatic, and prostate cancers.[105] Matsuzaki and colleagues used a machine learning approach with miRNAnomics to predict TOO for 13 cancer types from 7931 serum samples with 88% accuracy overall and 90% accuracy for precancer through stage II.[106]

The continued development of MCD tests represents a paradigm shift in cancer screening strategies by combining known biomarkers, high risk status of the patients, and AI to determine cancer risk and potential sites of origin. In alignment with the Cancer Moonshot[SM], NCI launched a new research network, the Cancer Screening Research Network (CSRN), that will assess the effectiveness of MCDs to prevent cancer-related deaths. Under CSRN's Vanguard study, NCI will begin enrolling 24,000 healthy people aged from 45 to 70 in 2024 to lay the foundation for future studies.[107]

Although MCD tests hold great promise to reduce cancer-related mortality, there is limited information and evidence on the clinical benefit especially in context of early-stage disease. Most MCD technologies perform poorly to detect early-stage disease with sensitivity varying between 40% and 50%.[108,109] Another clinical challenge is lack of clarity on how to diagnostically resolve and clinically manage a positive MCD test. MCD tests are considered adjuncts to current screening modalities, which currently are not efficient for all cancer types. Blood-based tests, in combination with subject characteristics, have the potential to make current screening more efficient by providing personalized screening schedules to individuals based on their own risk. For other less common cancers for which population-level screening is not practical, blood-based tests could identify individuals at sufficiently high risk to be screened for these cancers. However, the current candidate MCD technologies require rigorous investigation with respect to safety and effectiveness for reducing the morbidity and mortality associated with the cancers. To address these issues, careful assessment of the clinical utility of the assays by clinical trials through a well-established infrastructure may be essential.

FUTURE DIRECTIONS

The future holds promise for personalized risk assessment and inclusion of biomarkers that would have the potential to tailor screening according to risk and for other cancers to identify individuals for close monitoring. Improved screening for these cancers and effective evaluation of liquid biopsy-based tests with high specificity for a broader set of cancers, particularly for those for which screening modalities are not available, have the potential to significantly reduce cancer mortality.[110]

The process from the establishment of the diagnostic performance of a new biomarker to producing convincing evidence that population screening for the biomarker can reduce mortality may involve a sequence of well-organized phases: development of technically sound and systematically evaluated assay/s, promising performance of the assay/s in case versus control followed by prospectively screened population (intended-use population), screening in the intended-use population must lead to earlier diagnosis and, a more treatable point in the disease's natural history and lastly, the upgrading or stage shift should be translated into sustained mortality reduction in larger study cohorts.[111] The NCI's Early Detection Research Network (EDRN) is addressing some of these needs by providing an infrastructure that is essential for developing and validating biomarkers for early cancer detection.[112] EDRN has established the phases of biomarker development to specify criteria for progression from one phase to the next.[20] The mission of the NCI's EDRN is to discover, develop, and validate blood and tissue-based biomarkers and imaging methods to detect early-stage cancers and to translate these into clinical tests.[112,113] The EDRN is a highly collaborative program that consists of Biomarker Developmental Laboratories, Biomarker Reference Laboratories, Clinical Validation Centers, and a Data Management and Coordinating Center. EDRN has successfully completed several multicenter validation studies. Additionally, the EDRN has built biospecimen, including organ specific, reference sets, and informatics resources that are available to investigators both within and outside the EDRN.

In addition, AI methodologies including computational disease modeling have emerged as a successful tool for risk stratification and early cancer detection.[114] Many companies, academic centers, and government agencies are attempting to build databases to use data for risk prediction, identify patients for clinical trials, and develop drugs.[115] However, AI in general health care faces several challenges including ethical considerations, governance and data access, and security. Therefore, developing an ethically compliant framework for AI use in early cancer detection will be an important step. Since research on biomarkers is becoming more digitized and a vast amount of data are being collected through high dimensional omics and imaging technologies, sharing of such data has become paramount in leveraging methodologies and resources across scientific disciplines.

Overall, the early detection assay/s should demonstrate safety, accuracy, acceptability, cost-effectiveness, and reach in the general populations. Once these tests have been shown to reduce death from cancer, they need to be integrated in the health care system. Early detection should be accessible to all populations, particularly the groups with disproportionately high cancer mortality rates and should not lead to overdiagnosis and overtreatment. With the advancement in novel early detection technologies together with enhanced knowledge of cancer biology, we have an opportunity to translate these in early cancer detection to potentially reduce the cancer associated morbidity and mortality.

DISCLOSURE

The opinions expressed in this article are the authors' own and do not reflect the view of the National Institutes of Health, the Department of Health, and Human Services of the United States Government.

REFERENCES

1. Sung H, Ferlay J, Siegel RL, et al. Global Cancer Statistics 2020: GLOBOCAN Estimates of Incidence and Mortality Worldwide for 36 Cancers in 185 Countries. CA Cancer J Clin 2021;71:209–49.
2. Siegel RL, Miller KD, Wagle NS, et al. Cancer statistics, 2023. CA Cancer J Clin 2023;73:17–48.

3. Furlow B. US Government releases National Cancer Plan. Lancet Oncol 2023;24.

4. Howlader N, Noone AM, Krapcho M, et al. SEER Cancer Statistics Review, 1975-2018, National Cancer Institute. Bethesda, MD, based on November 2020 SEER data submission, posted to the SEER web site, 2021. Available at: https://seer.cancer.gov/csr/1975_2018/. Accessed April 2021.

5. SS PDW. National Cancer Institute's early detection research network: a model organization for biomarker research. Journal of the National Cancer Center 2023;3.

6. Blackford AL, Canto MI, Klein AP, et al. Recent Trends in the Incidence and Survival of Stage 1A Pancreatic Cancer: A Surveillance, Epidemiology, and End Results Analysis. J Natl Cancer Inst 2020;112:1162–9.

7. Schröder FH, Hugosson J, Roobol MJ, et al. Screening and prostate-cancer mortality in a randomized European study. N Engl J Med 2009;360:1320–8.

8. Frånlund M, Månsson M, Godtman RA, et al. Results from 22 years of Followup in the Göteborg Randomized Population-Based Prostate Cancer Screening Trial. J Urol 2022;208:292–300.

9. Wilt TJ, Jones KM, Barry MJ, et al. Follow-up of Prostatectomy versus Observation for Early Prostate Cancer. N Engl J Med 2017;377:132–42.

10. Andriole GL, Crawford ED, Grubb RL, et al. Mortality results from a randomized prostate-cancer screening trial. N Engl J Med 2009;360:1310–9.

11. Siegel RL, Giaquinto AN, Jemal A. Cancer statistics, 2024. CA A Cancer J Clin 2024;74:12–49.

12. Bokhorst LP, Zappa M, Carlsson SV, et al. Correlation between stage shift and differences in mortality in the European Randomized study of Screening for Prostate Cancer (ERSPC). BJU Int 2016;118:677–80.

13. USPST F, SJ C, AH K, et al. Screening for Cervical Cancer: US Preventive Services Task Force Recommendation Statement. JAMA 2018;320:674–86.

14. Stewart DB. Updated USPSTF Guidelines for Colorectal Cancer Screening: The Earlier the Better. JAMA Surg 2021;156:708–9.

15. USPST F, AH K, KW D, et al. Screening for Lung Cancer: US Preventive Services Task Force Recommendation Statement. JAMA 2021;325:962–70.

16. Siu AL, USPST F. Screening for Breast Cancer: U.S. Preventive Services Task Force Recommendation Statement. Ann Intern Med 2016;164:279–96.

17. Wolf AM, Wender RC, Etzioni RB, et al. American Cancer Society guideline for the early detection of prostate cancer: update 2010. CA Cancer J Clin 2010;60:70–98.

18. Henry NL, Hayes DF. Cancer biomarkers. Mol Oncol 2012;6:140–6.

19. Biomarkers Definitions Working Group. Biomarkers and surrogate endpoints: preferred definitions and conceptual framework. Clin Pharmacol Ther 2001;69:89–95.

20. Pepe MS, Etzioni R, Feng Z, et al. Phases of Biomarker Development for Early Detection of Cancer. JNCI: Journal of the National Cancer Institute 2001;93:1054–61.

21. Schiffman JD, Fisher PG, Gibbs P. Early detection of cancer: past, present, and future. Am Soc Clin Oncol Educ Book 2015;57–65.

22. Sprague BL, Arao RF, Miglioretti DL, et al. National performance benchmarks for modern diagnostic digital mammography: update from the Breast Cancer Surveillance Consortium. Radiology 2017;283:59–69.

23. Pinsky PF, Gierada DS, Black W, et al. Performance of Lung-RADS in the National Lung Screening Trial: a retrospective assessment. Annals of internal medicine 2015;162:485–91.
24. Croswell JM, Kramer BS, Kreimer AR, et al. Cumulative incidence of false-positive results in repeated, multimodal cancer screening. Ann Fam Med 2009;7:212–22.
25. Narayan A, Fischer A, Zhang Z, et al. Nationwide cross-sectional adherence to mammography screening guidelines: national behavioral risk factor surveillance system survey results. Breast Cancer Res Treat 2017;164:719–25.
26. Limmer K, LoBiondo-Wood G, Dains J. Predictors of cervical cancer screening adherence in the United States: a systematic review. Journal of the advanced practitioner in oncology 2014;5.
27. Daskalakis C, DiCarlo M, Hegarty S, et al. Predictors of overall and test-specific colorectal cancer screening adherence. Prev Med 2020;133.
28. Zahnd WE, Eberth JM. Lung Cancer Screening Utilization: A Behavioral Risk Factor Surveillance System Analysis. Am J Prev Med 2019;57:250–5.
29. Pinsky PF, Berg CD. Applying the National Lung Screening Trial eligibility criteria to the US population: what percent of the population and of incident lung cancers would be covered? J Med Screen 2012;19:154–6.
30. Fiscella K, Holt K, Meldrum S, et al. Disparities in preventive procedures: comparisons of self-report and Medicare claims data. BMC Health Serv Res 2006; 6:122.
31. Villarreal L, Méndez O, Salvans C, et al. Unconventional Secretion is a Major Contributor of Cancer Cell Line Secretomes. Mol Cell Proteomics 2013;12: 1046–60.
32. Srivastava S, Wagner PD, Hughes SK, et al. PreCancer Atlas: Present and Future. Cancer Prev Res 2023;16:379–84.
33. Hartmann LC, Degnim AC, Santen RJ, et al. Atypical hyperplasia of the breast–risk assessment and management options. N Engl J Med 2015;372:78–89.
34. Huck MB, Bohl JL. Colonic Polyps: Diagnosis and Surveillance. Clin Colon Rectal Surg 2016;29:296–305.
35. Distler M, Aust D, Weitz J, et al. Precursor lesions for sporadic pancreatic cancer: PanIN, IPMN, and MCN. BioMed Res Int 2014;2014:474905.
36. Caudill J, Thomas JE, Burkhart CG. The risk of metastases from squamous cell carcinoma of the skin. Int J Dermatol 2023;62:483–6.
37. Nasiell K, Nasiell M, Vaclavinkova V. Behavior of moderate cervical dysplasia during long-term follow-up. Obstet Gynecol 1983;61:609–14.
38. Merrick DT, Gao D, Miller YE, et al. Persistence of Bronchial Dysplasia Is Associated with Development of Invasive Squamous Cell Carcinoma. Cancer Prev Res 2016;96–104.
39. Kader T, Hill P, Rakha EA, et al. Atypical ductal hyperplasia: update on diagnosis, management, and molecular landscape. Breast Cancer Res 2018;20:39.
40. Corley DA, Jensen CD, Marks AR, et al. Variation of adenoma prevalence by age, sex, race, and colon location in a large population: implications for screening and quality programs. Clin Gastroenterol Hepatol 2013;11:172–80.
41. Peters MLB, Eckel A, Mueller PP, et al. Progression to pancreatic ductal adenocarcinoma from pancreatic intraepithelial neoplasia: Results of a simulation model. Pancreatology 2018;18:928–34.
42. Piquero-Casals J, Morgado-Carrasco D, Gilaberte Y, et al. Management Pearls on the Treatment of Actinic Keratoses and Field Cancerization. Dermatol Ther 2020;10:903–15.

43. Zynger DL, Yang X. High-grade prostatic intraepithelial neoplasia of the prostate: the precursor lesion of prostate cancer. Int J Clin Exp Pathol 2009;2: 327–38.

44. Marcus MW, Duffy SW, Devaraj A, et al. Probability of cancer in lung nodules using sequential volumetric screening up to 12 months: the UKLS trial. Thorax 2019;74:761–7.

45. Grimont A, Leach SD, Chandwani R. Uncertain Beginnings: Acinar and Ductal Cell Plasticity in the Development of Pancreatic Cancer. Cell Mol Gastroenterol Hepatol 2022;13:369–82.

46. Hong R, Koga Y, Bandyadka S, et al. Comprehensive generation, visualization, and reporting of quality control metrics for single-cell RNA sequencing data. Nat Commun 2022;13:1688. https://doi.org/10.1038/s41467-022-29212-9.

47. Strand SH, Rivero-Gutiérrez B, Houlahan KE, et al. Molecular classification and biomarkers of clinical outcome in breast ductal carcinoma in situ: Analysis of TBCRC 038 and RAHBT cohorts. Cancer Cell 2022;40:1521–36.e7.

48. RFA-CA-23-040: Pre-Cancer Atlas (PCA). Research Centers (U01 Clinical Trial Not Allowed). Available at: https://grants.nih.gov/grants/guide/rfa-files/RFA-CA-23-040.html. [Accessed 20 December 2023].

49. Maruvada P, Wang W, Wagner PD, et al. Biomarkers in molecular medicine: cancer detection and diagnosis. Biotechniques 2005;Suppl:9–15.

50. Yurgelun MB, Chenevix-Trench G, Lippman SM. Translating Germline Cancer Risk into Precision Prevention. Cell 2017;168:566–70.

51. Daly MB, Pal T, Maxwell KN, et al. NCCN Guidelines(R) Insights: Genetic/Familial High-Risk Assessment: Breast, Ovarian, and Pancreatic, Version 2.2024. J Natl Compr Canc Netw 2023;21:1000–10.

52. Kuchenbaecker KB, Hopper JL, Barnes DR, et al. Risks of Breast, Ovarian, and Contralateral Breast Cancer for BRCA1 and BRCA2 Mutation Carriers. JAMA 2017;317:2402–16.

53. Peltomaki P, Nystrom M, Mecklin JP, et al. Lynch Syndrome Genetics and Clinical Implications. Gastroenterology 2023;164:783–99.

54. FDA Grants First Marketing Authorization for a DNA Test to Assess Predisposition for Dozens of Cancer Types. 2023, FDA News Release.

55. Mitchell AC, Alford SC, Hunter SA, et al. Development of a Protease Biosensor Based on a Dimerization-Dependent Red Fluorescent Protein. ACS Chem Biol 2018;13:66–72.

56. Grant SA, Weilbaecher C, Lichlyter D. Development of a protease biosensor utilizing silica nanobeads. Sensor Actuator B Chem 2007;121:482–9.

57. Mac QD, Mathews DV, Kahla JA, et al. Non-invasive early detection of acute transplant rejection via nanosensors of granzyme B activity. Nat Biomed Eng 2019;3:281–91.

58. Kirkpatrick JD, Warren AD, Soleimany AP, et al. Urinary detection of lung cancer in mice via noninvasive pulmonary protease profiling. Sci Transl Med 2020;12: eaaw0262.

59. Hao L, Zhao RT, Welch NL, et al. CRISPR-Cas-amplified urinary biomarkers for multiplexed and portable cancer diagnostics. Nat Nanotechnol 2023;18: 798–807.

60. Xu D, Jalal SI, Sledge GW, et al. Small-molecule binding sites to explore protein-protein interactions in the cancer proteome. Mol Biosyst 2016;12:3067–87.

61. Niu P, Zhu J, Wei L, et al. Application of Fluorescent Probes in Reactive Oxygen Species Disease Model. Crit Rev Anal Chem 2022;1–36.

62. Lange J, Eddhif B, Tarighi M, et al. Volatile Organic Compound Based Probe for Induced Volatolomics of Cancers. Angew Chem Int Ed Engl 2019;58:17563–6.
63. Nandakumar A, Wei W, Siddiqui G, et al. Dynamic Protein Corona of Gold Nanoparticles with an Evolving Morphology. ACS Appl Mater Interfaces 2021;13: 58238–51.
64. Digiacomo L, Caputo D, Coppola R, et al. Efficient pancreatic cancer detection through personalized protein corona of gold nanoparticles. Biointerphases 2021;16:011010.
65. Wu T, Chen K, Lai W, et al. Bovine serum albumin-gold nanoclusters protein corona stabilized polystyrene nanoparticles as dual-color fluorescent nanoprobes for breast cancer detection. Biosens Bioelectron 2022;215:114575.
66. Segets D, Lucas JM, Klupp Taylor RN, et al. Determination of the Quantum Dot Band Gap Dependence on Particle Size from Optical Absorbance and Transmission Electron Microscopy Measurements. ACS Nano 2012;6:9021–32.
67. Winnik FM, Maysinger D. Quantum dot cytotoxicity and ways to reduce it. Acc Chem Res 2013;46:672–80.
68. Wang Y, Tang M. Dysfunction of various organelles provokes multiple cell death after quantum dot exposure. Int J Nanomedicine 2018;13:2729–42.
69. Liu J-H, Wang Y, Yan G-H, et al. Systematic Toxicity Evaluations of High-Performance Carbon "Quantum" Dots. J Nanosci Nanotechnol 2019;19:2130–7.
70. Zhao C, Song X, Liu Y, et al. Synthesis of graphene quantum dots and their applications in drug delivery. J Nanobiotechnol 2020;18:142.
71. Buszewska-Forajta M, Monedeiro F, Gołębiowski A, et al. Citric Acid as a Potential Prostate Cancer Biomarker Determined in Various Biological Samples. Metabolites 2022;12:268.
72. Rajalakshmi K, Deng T, Muthusamy S, et al. Prostate cancer biomarker citrate detection using triaminoguanidinium carbon dots, its applications in live cells and human urine samples. Spectrochim Acta Mol Biomol Spectrosc 2022;268: 120622.
73. Liu X, Braun GB, Qin M, et al. In vivo cation exchange in quantum dots for tumor-specific imaging. Nat Commun 2017;8:343.
74. Fang Y, Wolfson B, Godbey WT. Non-invasive detection of bladder cancer via expression-targeted gene delivery. J Gene Med 2017;19:366–75.
75. Kelly KJ, Wong J, Gönen M, et al. Human Trial of a Genetically Modified Herpes Simplex Virus for Rapid Detection of Positive Peritoneal Cytology in the Staging of Pancreatic Cancer. EBioMedicine 2016;7:94–9.
76. Aalipour A, Chuang H-Y, Murty S, et al. Engineered immune cells as highly sensitive cancer diagnostics. Nat Biotechnol 2019;37:531–9.
77. Panteli JT, Forkus BA, Van Dessel N, et al. Genetically modified bacteria as a tool to detect microscopic solid tumor masses with triggered release of a recombinant biomarker. Integr Biol 2015;7:423–34.
78. Danino T, Prindle A, Kwong GA, et al. Programmable probiotics for detection of cancer in urine. Sci Transl Med 2015;7:289ra84.
79. Cooper RM, Wright JA, Ng JQ, et al. Engineered bacteria detect tumor DNA. Science 2023;381:682–6.
80. National Cancer Institute. Definition of liquid biopsy - NCI Dictionary of Cancer Terms. Available at: https://www.cancer.gov/publications/dictionaries/cancer-terms/def/liquid-biopsy.
81. Caputo V, Ciardiello F, Corte CMD, et al. Diagnostic value of liquid biopsy in the era of precision medicine: 10 years of clinical evidence in cancer. Explor Target Antitumor Ther 2023;4:102–38.

82. Iakovlev AP, Erofeev AS, Gorelkin PV. Novel Pumping Methods for Microfluidic Devices: A Comprehensive Review. Biosensors 2022;12:956.

83. Zoupanou S, Volpe A, Primiceri E, et al. SMILE Platform: An Innovative Microfluidic Approach for On-Chip Sample Manipulation and Analysis in Oral Cancer Diagnosis. Micromachines 2021;12. https://doi.org/10.3390/mi12080885.

84. Kim HS, Chen Y-C, Nör F, et al. Endothelial-derived interleukin-6 induces cancer stem cell motility by generating a chemotactic gradient towards blood vessels. Oncotarget 2017;8:100339–52.

85. Yang C-Y, Brooks E, Li Y, et al. Detection of picomolar levels of interleukin-8 in human saliva by SPR. Lab Chip 2005;5:1017–23.

86. Park M-H, Reátegui E, Li W, et al. Enhanced Isolation and Release of Circulating Tumor Cells Using Nanoparticle Binding and Ligand Exchange in a Microfluidic Chip. J Am Chem Soc 2017;139:2741–9.

87. Lee H, Park C, Na W, et al. Precision cell-free DNA extraction for liquid biopsy by integrated microfluidics. npj Precis Onc 2020;4:1–10.

88. Radisic M, Loskill P. Beyond PDMS and Membranes: New Materials for Organ-on-a-Chip Devices. ACS Biomater Sci Eng 2021;7:2861–3.

89. Prabhakar P, Sen RK, Dwivedi N, et al. 3D-Printed Microfluidics and Potential Biomedical Applications. Frontiers in Nanotechnology 2021;3. Available at: https://www.frontiersin.org/articles/10.3389/fnano.2021.609355.

90. Moon S. Extending the Shelf-Life of Immunoassay-Based Microfluidic Chips through Freeze-Drying Sublimation Techniques. Sensors 2023;23:8524.

91. Lofton-Day C, Model F, Devos T, et al. DNA methylation biomarkers for blood-based colorectal cancer screening. Clin Chem. 2008;54:414–23.

92. Potter NT, Hurban P, White MN, et al. Validation of a Real-Time PCR–Based Qualitative Assay for the Detection of Methylated SEPT9 DNA in Human Plasma. Clin Chem 2014;60:1183–91.

93. Bluestar genomics presents positive results from validation study in pancreatic cancer detection at American pancreatic association (APA), Bluestar Genomics, Inc. News Release.

94. Lou PJ, Jacky Lam WK, Hsu WL, et al. Performance and Operational Feasibility of Epstein-Barr Virus-Based Screening for Detection of Nasopharyngeal Carcinoma: Direct Comparison of Two Alternative Approaches. J Clin Oncol 2023; 41:4257–66.

95. Cohen JD, Li L, Wang Y, et al. Detection and localization of surgically resectable cancers with a multi-analyte blood test. Science 2018;359:926–30.

96. Hinestrosa JP, Kurzrock R, Lewis JM, et al. Early-stage multi-cancer detection using an extracellular vesicle protein-based blood test. Commun Med 2022; 2:29.

97. Cristiano S, Leal A, Phallen J, et al. Genome-wide cell-free DNA fragmentation in patients with cancer. Nature 2019;570:385–9.

98. Luan Y, Zhong G, Li S, et al. A panel of seven protein tumour markers for effective and affordable multi-cancer early detection by artificial intelligence: a large-scale and multicentre case-control study. EClinicalMedicine 2023;61:102041.

99. Klein EA, Richards D, Cohn A, et al. Clinical validation of a targeted methylation-based multi-cancer early detection test using an independent validation set. Ann Oncol 2021;32:1167–77.

100. Lennon AM, Buchanan AH, Kinde I, et al. Feasibility of blood testing combined with PET-CT to screen for cancer and guide intervention. Science 2020;369: eabb9601.

101. Liu MC. Transforming the landscape of early cancer detection using blood tests-Commentary on current methodologies and future prospects. Br J Cancer 2021; 124:1475–7.
102. Nadauld LD, McDonnell CH, Beer TM, et al. The PATHFINDER Study: Assessment of the Implementation of an Investigational Multi-Cancer Early Detection Test into Clinical Practice. Cancers 2021;13:3501.
103. Ludwig N, Leidinger P, Becker K, et al. Distribution of miRNA expression across human tissues. Nucleic Acids Res 2016;44:3865–77.
104. Schwarzenbach H, Nishida N, Calin GA, et al. Clinical relevance of circulating cell-free microRNAs in cancer. Nat Rev Clin Oncol 2014;11:145–56.
105. Zhang A, Hu H. A Novel Blood-Based microRNA Diagnostic Model with High Accuracy for Multi-Cancer Early Detection. Cancers 2022;14:1450.
106. Matsuzaki J, Kato K, Oono K, et al. Prediction of tissue-of-origin of early stage cancers using serum miRNomes. JNCI Cancer Spectr 2023;7:pkac080.
107. Multicancer Detection Assays Promise to Improve Cancer Screening. But Do They Work? In: ASCO Daily News [Internet]. Available at: https://dailynews.ascopubs.org/do/10.1200/ADN.23.201572/full. [Accessed 19 December 2023].
108. Etzioni R, Gulati R, Weiss NS. Multicancer Early Detection: Learning From the Past to Meet the Future. J Natl Cancer Inst 2022;114:349–52.
109. Liu MC, Oxnard GR, Klein EA, et al. Sensitive and specific multi-cancer detection and localization using methylation signatures in cell-free DNA. Ann Oncol 2020;31:745–59.
110. Minasian LM, Pinsky P, Katki HA, et al. Study design considerations for trials to evaluate multicancer early detection assays for clinical utility. J Natl Cancer Inst 2022;115:250–7.
111. Etzioni R, Gulati R, Patriotis C, et al. Revisiting the standard blueprint for biomarker development to address emerging cancer early detection technologies. JNCI: Journal of the National Cancer Institute 2023;djad227. https://doi.org/10.1093/jnci/djad227.
112. Srivastava S, Wagner PD. The Early Detection Research Network: A National Infrastructure to Support the Discovery, Development, and Validation of Cancer Biomarkers. Cancer Epidemiol Biomarkers Prev 2020;29:2401–10.
113. National Cancer Institute. The early detection research network. Fifth report. National Institutes of Health; 2011. https://doi.org/10.32388/5F3KXD.
114. Kenner B, Chari ST, Kelsen D, et al. Artificial Intelligence and Early Detection of Pancreatic Cancer: 2020 Summative Review. Pancreas 2021;50:251–79.
115. Crichton DJ, Altinok A, Amos CI, et al. Cancer Biomarkers and Big Data: A Planetary Science Approach. Cancer Cell 2020;38:757–60.

Moving?

Make sure your subscription moves with you!

To notify us of your new address, find your **Clinics Account Number** (located on your mailing label above your name), and contact customer service at:

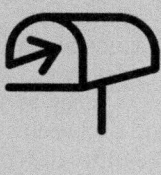

Email: journalscustomerservice-usa@elsevier.com

800-654-2452 (subscribers in the U.S. & Canada)
314-447-8871 (subscribers outside of the U.S. & Canada)

Fax number: 314-447-8029

Elsevier Health Sciences Division
Subscription Customer Service
3251 Riverport Lane
Maryland Heights, MO 63043

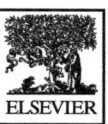

ELSEVIER

Printed and bound by CPI Group (UK) Ltd, Croydon, CR0 4YY

08/05/2025

01864751-0009